A GLOBAL IMPACT

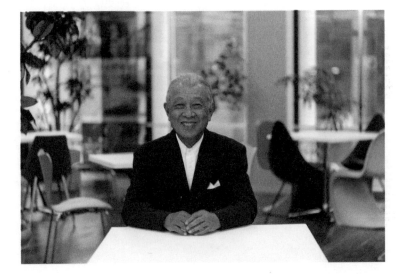

SHIGEKI SAKAMOTO
TAKAHIRO NANRI
(*Editors*)

A Global Impact

*Reflections on the Work of
Yohei Sasakawa, the WHO's Goodwill
Ambassador for Leprosy Elimination*

HURST & COMPANY, LONDON

First published in the United Kingdom in 2023 by
C. Hurst & Co. (Publishers) Ltd.,
New Wing, Somerset House, Strand, London, WC2R 1LA
© Shigeki Sakamoto, Takahiro Nanri and the Contributors, 2023
All rights reserved.

Distributed in the United States, Canada and Latin America by
Oxford University Press, 198 Madison Avenue, New York, NY 10016,
United States of America.

The right of Shigeki Sakamoto, Takahiro Nanri and the
Contributors to be identified as the authors of this
publication is asserted by them in accordance with the
Copyright, Designs and Patents Act, 1988.

Photo of Mr. Yohei Sasakawa: The Nippon Foundation.

A Cataloguing-in-Publication data record for this book
is available from the British Library.

ISBN: 9781805261292

This book is printed using paper from registered sustainable
and managed sources.

www.hurstpublishers.com

Printed in Great Britain by Bell and Bain Ltd, Glasgow

CONTENTS

CONTENTS

LIST OF FIGURES, MAPS AND TABLES

Figures

Maps

Tables

LIST OF CONTRIBUTORS

Shigeki Sakamoto is Professor Emeritus of International Law at Kobe University and President of the Center for Human Rights Education and Training, Tokyo. He was previously President of the Japanese Society of International Law and President of the Japanese Association of International Human Rights. As a member of the Advisory Committee of the UN Human Rights Council between 2008 and 2013, he drafted the document "Principles and guidelines for the elimination of discrimination against persons affected by leprosy and their family members". His research interests cover law of treaties, law of the sea, international human rights law and international dispute settlement.

Takahiro Nanri PhD is Executive Director of the Sasakawa Health Foundation previously Associate Professor, Faculty of Tourism and Community Studies, Atomi University. He is also Vice Chair of the Global Partnership for Zero Leprosy, a board member of the Sasakawa-India Leprosy Foundation, and Steering Committee Member, Japan Alliance on Global NTDs. He was previously Associate Professor, Faculty of Tourism and Community Studies, Atomi University, Program Advisor at The Nippon Foundation and Director of the Sasakawa Peace Foundation USA, among many other roles.

Artur Custódio Moreira de Sousa has been involved in voluntary health initiatives for many years. In 1984, he joined the

Movement for the Reintegration of Persons Affected by Hansen's Disease (MORHAN), Brazil. He has served as MORHAN's National Coordinator on multiple occasions, representing the movement in various organizations such as the National Council for the Rights of the Elderly, the National Council for the Rights of Persons with Disabilities, the National Health Council and the Intercultural Indigenous Health Commission. Currently, he holds a special advisory role in the General Coordination of Transmissible Diseases in Primary Health Care at the Brazilian Ministry of Health, and provides support in the national coordination of MORHAN.

Derek Lobo, Leprologist / Public Health Specialist, has devoted his entire professional career to treating and eliminating leprosy, and has a long association with Mr. Yohei Sasakawa. His leprosy-related work has included assignments in Mangalore, Dhanbad and Chennai in India; Addis Ababa and Harar, Ethiopia; in Dhaka, Bangladesh; and in the World Health Organization (WHO) Regional Office for South-East Asia, New Delhi. As a WHO consultant, he played a part in achieving the goal of eliminating leprosy as a public health problem in Bangladesh in 1998 and in India in 2005.

Tatsuya Tanami is Special Advisor and former Executive Director at The Nippon Foundation. Before joining the Foundation, Tanami worked at the International House of Japan, a private, non-profit organization based in Tokyo that promotes cultural exchange and intellectual cooperation between Japan, the US and other countries. Tanami is also a sitting board member of the Scandinavia-Japan Sasakawa Foundation, the Great Britain Sasakawa Foundation, the Fondation Franco-Japonaise Sasakawa, and the Sasakawa-India Leprosy Foundation. He is a graduate of Tokyo University of Foreign Studies and was a fellow at Wittenberg University in Ohio.

Marcos Virmond PhD is a professor on the medical course at the Bauru Faculty of Odontology, University of São Paulo (FOB-USP). Dr. Virmond also served as Director of the Instituto Lauro de Souza Lima, an international research centre for leprosy in Brazil, for 20 years. He is the former President of the International Leprosy Association (ILA) and of the Brazilian Leprosy Society (SBH), and has also acted as a consultant for the Pan American Health Organization (PAHO) and the WHO. Dr. Virmond's publications cover areas such as rehabilitation, surgery, epidemiology and the prevention of disabilities, and he is an associated editor of *Hansen's Disease: A Complete Clinical Guide*.

The Nippon Foundation

The Nippon Foundation (TNF), founded by Ryoichi Sasakawa, has been providing funding to leprosy-related initiatives since 1967. In addition to providing the majority of funding for SHF and the WHO Goodwill Ambassador's activities, TNF has been the main donor to the WHO's Global Leprosy Programme since 1975. www.nippon-foundation.or.jp

Sasakawa Health Foundation

Sasakawa Health Foundation (SHF) was co-founded in 1974 by Yohei's father, Ryoichi Sasakawa, and Morizo Ishidate, a pharmacologist who was the first person to synthesize a drug treatment for leprosy in Japan. SHF is committed to a public health approach and collaborates with a wide range of stakeholders in order to address interrelated medical and social issues. www.shf.or.jp

Sasakawa Leprosy (Hansen's Disease) Initiative

Sasakawa Leprosy (Hansen's Disease) Initiative is a strategic alliance formed in 2020 between WHO Goodwill Ambassador for Leprosy Elimination Yohei Sasakawa, The Nippon Foundation and Sasakawa Health Foundation for the purpose of achieving zero leprosy: a world free from all forms of suffering associated with the disease. Leprosy Programs of both The Nippon Foundation and Sasakawa Health Foundation have been merged under the Initiative. sasakawaleprosyinitiative.org

FOREWORD

MR. YOHEI SASAKAWA'S 20TH ANNIVERSARY AS WHO GOODWILL AMBASSADOR FOR LEPROSY ELIMINATION

Tedros Adhanom Ghebreyesus, Director-General,
World Health Organization

Leprosy, or Hansen's disease, has afflicted humanity for millennia, as reflected in the literature, art and faith traditions of many countries. Leprosy has been a source of suffering for so long that it is perhaps difficult to imagine a world without it. But it is an attainable goal, and one that is coming closer, thanks to the dedication of people such as Mr. Yohei Sasakawa.

Mr. Sasakawa was first appointed Special Ambassador for the Global Alliance for the Elimination of Leprosy (GAEL) by WHO Director-General Dr. Gro Harlem Brundtland in 2001, then WHO Goodwill Ambassador for Leprosy Elimination in 2004. In the two decades since being appointed Ambassador, Mr. Sasakawa's commitment and dedication to the fight against leprosy and the health of neglected populations has been key to progress against leprosy and other diseases. In his time as Goodwill Ambassador,

Mr. Sasakawa has visited more than 100 countries, meeting with affected communities, presidents and prime ministers, kings and queens, business and religious leaders and many more, to champion the cause of leprosy elimination. Since 1975, The Nippon Foundation and the Sasakawa Health Foundation have been the principal donors to the WHO Global Leprosy Programme.

Mr. Sasakawa has been instrumental in the fight not just against leprosy, but against the stigma, discrimination and social exclusion that people with leprosy have faced throughout history. Unlike some diseases, which are transient, until recently people with leprosy were defined by it for the remainder of their lives. Despite being such an ancient disease, leprosy has attracted relatively little investment in research and development, and did not benefit as much as other diseases from the scientific and technological revolution of the twentieth and twenty-first centuries. Many aspects of its epidemiology remain elusive.

However, the advent of multidrug therapy (MDT) in the early 1980s was a major step towards the goal of leprosy elimination, by making it possible to cure patients and curtail the risk of onward transmission, enabling people affected by leprosy to rejoin their families and communities, and helping to mitigate the stigma and discrimination they often face. For many years these life-saving and life-changing medicines were provided free of charge to patients thanks to a generous donation by The Nippon Foundation.

As we celebrate twenty years of Mr. Sasakawa's appointment as WHO Goodwill Ambassador, on behalf of the whole WHO family I offer my deep gratitude and respect to Mr. Sasakawa for his unwavering commitment to, and solidarity with, people with leprosy around the world. I look forward to his continued support and our continued partnership as we work together towards the dream of eliminating leprosy.

1

TOWARDS A LEPROSY-FREE WORLD

THE PIONEERING ACTIVITIES OF MR. YOHEI SASAKAWA

Shigeki Sakamoto

Introduction

The year 2021 marked the twentieth anniversary of the appointment of Mr. Yohei Sasakawa, chairman of the Nippon Foundation, as the World Health Organization Goodwill Ambassador for Leprosy Elimination.[1] Dr. Tedros Adhanom Ghebreyesus, Director-General of the World Health Organization (WHO), said, "We are all thankful for the contribution Mr. Sasakawa has made to leprosy control programs in many countries. We can now harvest the fruits of his relentless efforts as the leprosy epidemic is slowly but surely fading away globally."[2]

As Director-General Tedros remarked, in discussing the current positive results achieved by efforts to eliminate leprosy, the activities of Mr. Yohei Sasakawa are an essential element. In April 2017, in honour of Mr. Sasakawa's contribution to the elimination of leprosy, the WHO, at the Global Partners' Meeting on Neglected Tropical Diseases held in Geneva under its auspices, awarded him the WHO Gold Medal.[3] Then, in February 2019, the government of India conferred the 2018 Gandhi Peace Prize on Mr. Sasakawa, in recognition of his contributions to the elimination of leprosy.[4]

These honours were in recognition of the work that Mr. Sasakawa has done over the past half century, including making over 200 visits to over 100 countries since becoming the WHO Goodwill Ambassador for Leprosy Elimination to convey the message that leprosy is not an incurable disease but in fact one that can be cured, and conducting a wide range of activities in support of efforts to stamp out prejudice and discrimination towards persons affected by leprosy and their family members.[5]

This chapter reflects on Mr. Yohei Sasakawa's leprosy elimination activities up until now, considers the pioneering aspect of his approach, and argues that the methods he has used to tackle leprosy issues can serve as a model for future efforts to combat new infectious diseases. This is because he has adopted a human rights approach to leprosy that will be fundamental in the fight against infectious diseases—not only COVID-19—that may arise in the twenty-first century.

Mr. Sasakawa first became aware of the tragic reality for sufferers of leprosy in 1965, when he accompanied his father, Mr. Ryoichi Sasakawa, to a leprosy treatment centre in South Korea.[6] Since then, Mr. Sasakawa has continued his father's work and tackled leprosy issues for more than fifty years. The uniqueness of his approach lies in the comprehensive stance he has taken in addressing both aspects of the leprosy issue: the medical aspect of eliminating leprosy and the social aspect of stamping out prejudice and discrimination against those affected by leprosy and their family members, and restoring their dignity as a human rights issue.[7] Considering that both public health and human rights share the same purpose of promoting and protecting the personal rights and well-being of all human beings, one can call this a natural approach.

Mr. Sasakawa's approach anticipates some of the methods we are currently using to achieve the seventeen international Sustainable Development Goals established by the United Nations (UN), which I would like to identify in this paper.

TOWARDS A LEPROSY-FREE WORLD

On 25 September 2015 the UN General Assembly (UNGA) adopted "Transforming our world: the 2030 Agenda for Sustainable Development" and established Sustainable Development Goals (SDGs) to take the place of the Millennium Development Goals (MDGs) of the 2000 to 2015 period. The UN established seventeen goals and 169 specific targets to be achieved in the period 2016 to 2030 to transform the world, as well as 232 indicators to specifically measure progress towards those targets.[8] Although based on the achievement of the eight MDGs, these measures also tackle unfinished challenges. In contrast to the MDGs, whose eight international goals were set exclusively for developing countries, the SDGs set seventeen international goals for all countries, developing and developed, including goals relating to global issues such as climate change.

The 2030 Agenda is a UN General Assembly Resolution, and is not legally binding, to avoid a situation where non-parties to a legally binding treaty could take the position that the common interests of those bound by the treaty are not their own interests. Instead, an UNGA Resolution has a legal structure that encourages the cooperation of all member states. Moreover, one of the advantages of employing this legal form is that, in order to achieve the SDGs, there is a need to establish cooperative goals not only for countries but for everyone on Earth, including diverse stakeholders such as corporations and civil society. Being in the form of an UNGA Resolution makes this possible.

Furthermore, the 2030 Agenda underlines the importance of partnership, stating:

> We are determined to mobilize the means required to implement this Agenda through a revitalised Global Partnership for Sustainable Development, based on a spirit of strengthened global solidarity, focused in particular on the needs of the poorest and most vulnerable and with the participation of all countries, all stakeholders and all people.[9]

Mr. Sasakawa's leprosy elimination activities first focused on the poorest and most vulnerable people suffering from leprosy in developing countries.[10] Observing the situation in developing countries with unsatisfactory access to medical services, Mr. Sasakawa provided for the free distribution of effective drugs in the form of multidrug therapy (MDT) for the five-year period between 1995 and 1999, to ensure that the drugs reached patients, no matter how remote their area.[11] As a result, even without going to specialized hospitals or treatment facilities, leprosy patients were able to receive medical services at general hospitals. This can be seen as anticipating the idea behind the COVAX Facility, co-led by the WHO and international organizations such as the Coalition for Epidemic Preparedness Innovations (CEPI) and Gavi, working on vaccination in developing countries, in which vaccines for the novel coronavirus (nCoV) are considered an international public good. In this, we can see a precedent for the inclusivity of the SDGs' "Leave No One Behind" slogan.

Further, we can see examples of good practice of partnership in the private sector in Mr. Sasakawa's activities as a Goodwill Ambassador for Leprosy Elimination. Mr. Sasakawa, in conjunction with World Leprosy Day, has actively collaborated with the medical world, the legal community, the business sector, politicians, labour unions, organizations of persons with disabilities and others. Since 2006, he has issued an annual "Global Appeal to End Stigma and Discrimination against Persons Affected by Leprosy". This is a clear example of the kind of global partnership promoted by the SDGs.

Moreover, an important feature of Mr. Sasakawa's activities is that he is not simply creating armchair theories towards achieving a leprosy-free world, but rather is himself tirelessly working towards that goal. He has personally travelled to leprosy treatment centres in the jungles of leprosy-endemic countries, such as Malawi and the Central African Republic, in support of leprosy elimination, truly reflecting the Leave No One Behind mindset espoused by the SDGs.[12]

Mr. Sasakawa has told sufferers of leprosy here and elsewhere, who had thought of leprosy as an incurable disease, that nowadays leprosy can in fact be cured using MDT. Unfortunately, however, prejudice and discrimination against persons affected by leprosy and their families remain throughout the world, both in developed and developing countries. Mr. Sasakawa has dedicated his life to these efforts to eliminate such prejudice and discrimination. There are many lessons to be learned in overcoming the current COVID-19 pandemic from Mr. Sasakawa's past measures regarding leprosy.

1. COVID-19 and human rights

On 30 January 2020, the WHO declared COVID-19 a Public Health Emergency of International Concern (PHEIC).[13] Against this background, on 23 April, António Guterres, UN Secretary-General, released a paper called "COVID-19 and Human Rights". In this he stated: "The COVID-19 pandemic is a public health emergency—but it is far more. It is an economic crisis. A social crisis. And a human crisis that is fast becoming a human rights crisis."[14] In a similar vein, the view that leprosy is not only a public health issue but also a human rights issue can be seen in Mr. Sasakawa's leprosy activities, as mentioned earlier.

On 29 June 2020, the WHO Director-General said: "the hard reality is: this is not even close to being over".[15] Indeed, the increase in COVID-19 infection through the emergence of the Delta variant in India and the Omicron variant in South Africa, has led to worldwide infection, and, as of mid-2023, there is still no end in sight.

In September 2020, UN Secretary-General Guterres said that the effects of the pandemic required a coordinated global response which included making vaccines accessible for every individual, regardless of their wealth, gender or legal immigration position, in order to save the future of the economy and society.[16]

Mr. Sasakawa's approach to leprosy, in particular his supplying MDT free of charge, was implemented based on the same way of thinking.

Of course, COVID-19 infections have the greatest effect on vulnerable people. This point was indicated in the joint press release issued on 31 March 2020 by the Office of the UN High Commissioner for Human Rights (OHCHR), the International Organization for Migration (IOM), the UN High Commissioner for Refugees (UNHCR) and the WHO. Along with indicating that "everyone has a risk of becoming infected by this virus, but people who are forced to move, including refugees, those with no nationality, and many emigrants suffer from a higher risk", the document also says:

> More than ever, as COVID-19 poses a global threat to our collective humanity, our primary focus should be on the preservation of life, regardless of status. This crisis demands a coherent, effective international approach that leaves no-one behind. At this crucial moment we all need to rally around a common objective, fighting this deadly virus.[17]

As Ms. Michelle Bachelet, then UN High Commissioner for Human Rights, said in her report to the 44th session of the Human Rights Council on 30 June 2020, there is a need to "ensure that human rights are at the heart of the response to the pandemic", while it goes without saying that "we must all acknowledge that human rights are critical to the recovery".[18] For the elimination of COVID-19, vaccinations must be carried out in both developed and developing countries in a manner that "leaves no one behind", as stated in the SDGs.

As noted in a statement issued by forty-three UN Special Rapporteurs, including the Special Rapporteur on the right to health, "Everyone, without exception, has the right to life-saving interventions." They went on: "When the vaccine for COVID-19 comes, it should be provided without discrimination. Meanwhile, as it is still to come, the human rights-based approach is already known as another effective pathway in the prevention of major public health threats."[19]

We must not forget this. Today we are seeing the reality that the more vaccine inequality continues, the more COVID-19 variants will spread. We must not forget the principle that "until everyone is safe, no one is safe".[20]

In the case of leprosy, there are differences from COVID-19. Leprosy has low infectiousness, and more than 95% of people exposed to the bacteria that cause leprosy do not develop the disease. Accordingly, rather than vaccines, more energy has been expended into treatments for leprosy.[21] In other regards, however, the two diseases do share similarities. In the same manner as the COVAX Facility, the international framework that facilitates the provision of vaccines to developing countries, MDT treatment for leprosy was offered free of charge to developing countries.

2. Measures in response to leprosy as an infectious disease

(i) Approaching the WHO

An approach to the WHO to eliminate leprosy was made by Mr. Ryoichi Sasakawa, the father of Mr. Yohei Sasakawa, in 1975. At the time, leprosy was considered a "neglected disease" even by the WHO. Mr. Ryoichi Sasakawa, then chair of the Japanese Shipbuilding Industry Foundation (JSIF)—which would become the Nippon Foundation in 1988—offered to provide US$1 million dollars to help countries in Africa that were suffering from leprosy. Dr. Halfdan T. Mahler, Director-General of the WHO at the time, accepted this offer from the Nippon Foundation, and promised to once again treat leprosy as a serious problem. Subsequently, with the approval of Mr. Ryoichi Sasakawa, half of the funds were used for the eradication of smallpox in Ethiopia and Somalia, something the WHO was focused on at the time.[22] Five years later, in 1980, the WHO declared that smallpox had been eradicated from the world.

This provision of funds resulted in increased interest in leprosy within the WHO and subsequently became a major cornerstone of leprosy elimination activities promoted by the Nippon Foundation in conjunction with the WHO. These actions were to be continued by Mr. Yohei Sasakawa, the son of Mr. Ryoichi Sasakawa.

(ii) Multidrug therapy (MDT)—a game-changer

In the 1970s, with the emergence of a type of leprosy that was resistant to dapsone (DDS), a drug used to treat leprosy, there was an urgent need to rethink ways to control the disease. In 1978, joint chemotherapy research was begun in South Korea, Thailand and the Philippines, and a start was made on empirical research on MDT.[23] This research continued until 1988, by which time the optimal dosage, duration and efficacy of MDT had been confirmed in all three countries and in Japan.[24]

7

Then, in October 1981, the WHO invited close to forty experts to Geneva, where it held a research meeting on prevention of the antibiotic-resistant bacteria that had become an obstacle in leprosy treatment, and agreed that leprosy patients should be treated with a combination of three drugs (rifampicin, clofazimine and dapsone).[25] Of these MDT drugs, the one that is considered most effective is the antibiotic rifampicin.[26] In March of the following year, 1982, the WHO released a report on MDT.[27] Since then, MDT has been promoted worldwide. As a result, the focus of measures against leprosy changed to speedily and effectively providing MDT to developing countries, which include many leprosy-endemic countries. In fact, in 1985, 5.3 million leprosy patients received MDT, and by 1991 the number of patients had dropped to 3.1 million.[28]

As a result of the significant therapeutic benefits of MDT, the WHO positioned this as a historical opportunity to actively implement a leprosy treatment initiative. The resolution on leprosy that was adopted at the 44th World Health Assembly in May 1991, declared "WHO's commitment to continuing to promote the use of all control measures including multidrug therapy together with case-finding in order to attain the global elimination of leprosy as a public health problem by the year 2000".[29] At that time, "elimination" of leprosy was defined as a prevalence of less than one leprosy patient per 10,000 population.[30] This was based on the assumption that if prevalence could be lowered to less than one case per 10,000 population, then each country would somehow manage to cope with it through its own health care system, given that leprosy has a low rate of infection.

In other words, this meant that, if this goal could be achieved, leprosy would no longer be a "major public health problem". At the same time, this method of setting in advance a numerical value as the "elimination goal" was a unique approach that had never been tried before.[31] This method of establishing indicators for the achievement of goals was adopted in the MDGs and SDGs, and can be seen as one of the early models for setting specific targets and indicators to measure concrete progress toward those targets that are used for the SDGs.[32]

In July 1994, an International Conference on the Elimination of Leprosy as a Public Health Problem was held in Hanoi, Vietnam, under the joint auspices of the WHO and the Sasakawa Health Foundation. The purpose of this conference, which was attended by delegates from twenty-eight countries that had yet to achieve elimination, experts and NGOs, was to reconfirm the above-mentioned WHO resolution ("global elimination of leprosy as a public health problem by the year 2000") and to bolster the commitment of the twenty-eight countries. [33]

On this occasion, Mr. Sasakawa made the offer to provide the sum of US$10 million annually over a period of five years, for a total of US$50 million, to the WHO to supply MDT to health facilities, which was vital in the effort to eliminate leprosy by the year 2000. [34] As a result of this offer, measures for the elimination of leprosy in countries where the disease was still endemic suddenly became more concrete. Moreover, the Hanoi Declaration that was unanimously adopted at the conference stated that

> intensive and sustained efforts are still required to bring about elimination by the target date (the year 2000), and that national authorities, international bodies, donor agencies, national and international nongovernmental organizations and health professionals working in the field of leprosy must all step up their commitment to attain this goal. [35]

The free supply of MDT relieved governments of developing countries of the financial burden of buying MDT drugs, while at the same time allowing them to allocate budgets for health workers and social workers, as well as for awareness-raising activities on treatment. [36] This measure of Mr. Sasakawa's is a good example of a partnership in which the private sector cooperates when a state is unable to do something on its own, and has great pioneering significance. By 2010, all countries except Brazil and some small-island states with a population below 1 million had achieved the level of leprosy elimination as defined by the WHO. It is certain that Mr. Sasakawa's provision of medicines free of charge contributed to largely resolving the issue of leprosy as a public health problem. However, another aspect of leprosy—the discrimination and prejudice towards those who are affected by leprosy and their family members—continued as before in many countries.

In the period from 1985 to 2008, it is estimated that more than 15 million leprosy patients recovered as a result of the use of MDT. In fact, while in 1985 there were 122 countries that had not yet eliminated leprosy as a public health problem, by 2010 only Brazil and some small island states with a population below 1 million had yet to do so. It is said that the number of new cases dropped from 5.4 million in 1985 to 250,000 in 2008.

In the decade leading up to the COVID-19 pandemic, numbers of new cases had been declining very slowly, approaching the 200,000 mark, but with the subsequent disruption to leprosy services caused by the pandemic, the impact on case numbers will need to be assessed. [37]

(iii) The formation of the Global Alliance for the Elimination of Leprosy (GAEL)

In November 1999, the 3rd International Conference for the Elimination of Leprosy was held in Abidjan, Ivory Coast. At this conference, countries where the elimination of leprosy according to the WHO definition was considered difficult to achieve were identified, and concrete countermeasures were discussed. Also, a new international alliance called the Global Alliance for the Elimination of Leprosy (GAEL) was formed to disrupt the status quo, and the target year for the elimination of leprosy was pushed back to 2005. [38] Even though the goal had not been reached by the original deadline, the approach of resetting the deadline was useful. In fact, the first MDG goal, "Eradicate extreme poverty and hunger", was not achieved between 2000 and 2015, but was carried over as SDG Goal 1, "End poverty", for the period 2016 to 2030.

The members of the new alliance comprised the governments of the twelve countries most affected by the disease, the WHO, the International Federation of Anti-Leprosy Associations (ILEP), the Nippon Foundation, the Sasakawa Health Foundation, Novartis and the Novartis Foundation. Mr. Sasakawa, chair of the Nippon Foundation, indicated support to the extent of US$24 million from

2000 to 2005 for activities for the elimination of leprosy. Subsequently, the Novartis Foundation indicated that it would continue the provision of MDT free of charge.[39] The first GAEL meeting was held in January 2001 in New Delhi, India. There, the Delhi Declaration "to eliminate leprosy from every country by the year 2005" was adopted.[40]

However, although the world was moving towards the resolution of leprosy as a public health issue in this way, stigma and discrimination towards people affected by leprosy and their family members remained in developed and developing countries alike. One characteristic of issues around leprosy is the fact that such prejudice and discrimination exist in all countries, regardless of religion, culture or political and economic system.

When the WHO, as a UN agency, addresses leprosy as a public health problem, consideration of human rights is also a top priority. Yet it is fair to say that before Mr. Sasakawa's intervention, it was not necessarily a generally held view that this was an issue to be handled by other UN agencies that deal with human rights issues, namely, the UN Commission on Human Rights (at the time) and later the UN Human Rights Council.

3. Measures for leprosy as a human rights issue

(i) Approach to the UN Commission on Human Rights

In October 2001, at the 5th Forum 2000, Mr. Yohei Sasakawa, chair of the Nippon Foundation, who was also the chair of this forum, gave a report on "Human rights issues in relation to leprosy". Forum 2000 was an international conference that started in Prague, the Czech Republic in 1997, and was founded by the late Václav Havel, former president of the Czech Republic; Professor Elie Wiesel of Boston University, a recipient of the Nobel Peace Prize; and Mr. Yohei Sasakawa. The objective of this forum was for world leaders in a range of fields to seek resolution measures in regard to issues of common concern to humanity, such as ethnic issues, religious disputes, population matters and environmental concerns. The revelation by Mr. Sasakawa of the cruel discrimination related to leprosy had a strong impact on the participants and many become aware of "leprosy as a human rights issue" as a result of this conference. At the same time, it led to activities to confront leprosy as a human rights issue, including an approach to the UN Commission on Human Rights.

Mr. Sasakawa's approach to the UN began in July 2003. As well as having discussions with Dr. Bertrand Ramcharan, then the Acting High Commissioner for Human Rights and Assistant Secretary-General of the UN, and Professor Paul Hunt, Special Rapporteur on "Health and Human Rights" to the UN Commission on Human Rights, Mr. Sasakawa also held an explanatory meeting for staff members of the Office of the High Commissioner for Human Rights (OHCHR).[41] Further, during the term of the 55th UN Sub-Commission on the Promotion and Protection of Human Rights (at the time), as well as setting up a photography exhibition in the conference hall lobby of the Palais des Nations (UN Office) in Geneva, he organized a seminar of persons affected by leprosy and NGO representatives, as a side event.[42]

In March 2004, at the plenary meeting of the 60th session of the UN Commission on Human Rights, based on Resolution 1996/31 of the UN Economic and Social Council, utilizing the Nippon Foundation's position as an NGO with consultative status to the Economic and Social Council,[43] Mr. Sasakawa commented on "leprosy and discrimination". Mr. Sasakawa's passionate approach led to a resolution at the 56th session of the Sub-Commission on the Promotion and Protection of Human Rights to conduct an official survey on the issue of "discrimination against leprosy victims and their family members".[44]

On 5 August 2005, continuing on from the previous year, Mr. Sasakawa was again given the opportunity to speak at the 57th session of the Sub-Commission on the Promotion and Protection of Human Rights. On this occasion, four persons affected by leprosy from India, Ghana and Nepal were also provided with the opportunity to speak. Before that, a second Sub-Commission Resolution was passed and, under the discussion topic "the prevention of discrimination and protection of minorities", Professor Yozo Yokota, a member of the Sub-Commission, was asked by the Sub-Commission to provide his preliminary working report related to the issue of "discrimination against persons affected by leprosy and their family members" to the committee of the 57th meeting.[45] In the preliminary working report submitted to the committee in July 2005, Professor Yokota said:

> The treatment that leprosy patients and their family members have experienced from governments, local societies, schools, religious groups, etc., as well as other organs, involves serious violations of human rights. For a long period, leprosy patients and their families have been discriminated against in marriage and social activities. This type of discrimination exists even today in every corner of the globe.[46]

For much of the long history of humanity, leprosy was incurable. It was also mistakenly thought to be highly contagious. As a result, both sufferers from leprosy and those who had recovered were alienated and feared. There is a need to eradicate the deep-rooted discriminatory practices towards those affected by leprosy and their family members, which exist everywhere throughout the world.

The persistent lobbying activities of Mr. Sasakawa at the UN led to a shared recognition among states at the UN Commission on Human Rights that leprosy is a human rights issue. At this point, the Commission, which had been criticized for having become extremely politicized, was reorganized and replaced by the UN Human Rights Council (UNHRC)—newly established by UNGA in March 2006—and the Council resumed work on the topic.

(ii) Adoption of the "Principles and Guidelines" by the UN Human Rights Council

On 18 June 2008, Resolution 8/13 on elimination of discrimination against persons affected by leprosy and their family members, co-sponsored by fifty-nine countries including Japan (of which thirty-one were member states of the UNHRC), was adopted unanimously at the 8th session of the UN Human Rights Council. This resolution "affirms that persons affected by leprosy and their family members should be treated as individuals with dignity and are entitled to all basic human rights and fundamental freedoms under customary international law, relevant conventions and national constitutions and laws" (para. 1) and "Requests the Office of the United Nations High Commissioner for Human Rights to include the issue of discrimination against persons affected by leprosy and their family members as an important matter in its human rights education and awareness raising activities" (para. 3). In the same resolution, it also said that it "Requests the Human Rights Council Advisory Committee … [to] formulate a draft set of principles and guidelines for the elimination of discrimination against persons affected by leprosy and their family members, and to submit it to the Council for its consideration by September 2009" (para. 5).[47]

On receipt of this resolution, the Human Rights Council Advisory Committee, at its first meeting in August 2008, designated the author of this chapter, Professor Shigeki Sakamoto, as the Rapporteur for the "principles and guidelines for the elimination of discrimination against persons affected by leprosy and their family members".[48] Based on the above-mentioned Human Rights Council resolution, on 15 January 2009, a consultation was held in Geneva under the auspices of the Office of the United Nations High Commissioner for Human Rights (OHCHR). The approximately forty participants included representatives of national governments and NGOs, as well as persons affected by leprosy, who talked of the realities and their own experiences of discrimination.[49]

At the second meeting of the Human Rights Council Advisory Committee, from 26 to 30 January 2009, the author, as Rapporteur, proposed a basic policy, which was supported by the Advisory Committee, that in the principles to be developed, persons affected by leprosy should be considered as subjects of rights and that actions to be taken by each country to eliminate discrimination should be clearly stated as guidelines.

The Rapporteur stated that in order to eliminate discrimination against persons affected by leprosy, the issue of leprosy should be considered as a social problem, and that a social approach should be adopted to guarantee the rights of persons affected by leprosy and their family members and to prohibit discrimination against them.[50]

Finally, at the fifth meeting, held in August 2010, an amended version of the "principles and guidelines" proposed by Professor Sakamoto was adopted.[51] Then, on 30 September 2010, in UNHRC Resolution 15/10, appreciation was expressed for the principles and guidelines for the elimination of discrimination against persons affected by leprosy and their family members that the Advisory Committee had submitted to the UNHRC, and the resolution was unanimously adopted.[52] Shortly afterwards, on 21 December 2010, the resolution was jointly proposed at the UNGA by eighty-four countries, including Japan, and adopted unanimously. It noted with appreciation the principles and guidelines for the elimination of discrimination against persons affected by leprosy and their family members, and encouraged governments, relevant UN bodies and national human rights organizations, as well as all relevant actors in society, to give due consideration to them.[53]

At the time of the adoption of this resolution, Brazil was the only country that had not yet achieved the elimination of leprosy as a public health problem. However, even in countries that had, persons affected by leprosy continued, as before, to be the targets of severe prejudice and discrimination. Simply because resolutions to abolish discrimination had been adopted by the Human Rights Council and the UNGA, did not mean that all the prejudice and discrimination towards persons affected by leprosy and their families immediately disappeared.

Mr. Sasakawa, believing that the major challenge was to make the "principles and guidelines" known to as many people as possible, decided to hold a series of international symposiums on "leprosy and human rights". Starting with Rio de Janeiro, Brazil, in January 2012, he organized these events in New Delhi, India (2012), Addis Ababa, Ethiopia (2013), Rabat, Morocco (2014), and lastly in Geneva, Switzerland, in 2015. At the final symposium, recommendations for following up the UN resolutions and for action plans compiled based on discussions at previous symposiums, were presented.[54]

However, Mr. Sasakawa's persistence and ability to take action did not stop there. Seeing the need for a study by the UN Human

Rights Council Advisory Committee to review the implementation of the principles and guidelines, he lobbied governments, leading to the adoption in July 2015 by the UN Human Rights Council of the new Resolution 29/5.[55] On receipt of this, at the 15th session of the Advisory Committee, a working group of seven members was formed, with Mr. Kaoru Obata as the chair and Mr. Imeru Tamrat Yigezu as the Rapporteur.

Considering that when the author of this chapter became the Rapporteur of the "principles and guidelines" the working group had not been formed and had to work independently, there was a growing understanding of and interest in this issue within the Advisory Committee. Mr. Yigezu worked vigorously, submitting a preliminary report in February 2016[56] and a progress report in July 2016, in which he recommended promoting awareness and dissemination of the principles and guidelines at a national level, and that a specific and dedicated mechanism be established at the international level to follow up, monitor and report on progress made by countries at the national level towards effective implementation of the principles and guidelines.[57]

Seeing the way that countries were hesitating to establish a specific and dedicated mechanism to monitor the implementation of the principles and guidelines based on Mr. Yigezu's recommendations, Mr. Sasakawa intensified his efforts to reach out to the Japanese government and other governments, believing that the appointment of a Special Rapporteur was the best way to follow up on the principles and guidelines.

These efforts bore fruit in June 2017, when the UN Human Rights Council passed a resolution to appoint a Special Rapporteur on elimination of discrimination against persons affected by leprosy for a three-year term, to follow up on progress made and measures taken by states for the effective implementation of the principles and guidelines, and to engage in dialogue and consultation with states and other relevant stakeholders to promote good practice in the realization of the rights of persons affected by leprosy and their family members.[58]

As a result of this initiative, in November 2017 Ms. Alice Cruz was named as the Special Rapporteur from among eleven outstanding candidates.[59] Subsequently, through a new resolution of the UNHRC on July 2020,[60] her term was extended for a further three years. During this period, Ms. Cruz has actively pursued research and dialogue with countries to ensure the effective implementation of the principles and guidelines and dialogues with countries, and submitted to the UNHRC and the UNGA three reports: one on stereotyping and structural violence against women and children affected by leprosy,[61] and the other two on her visits to Brazil and Japan.[62] Then, in September 2021, Ms. Cruz presented a report titled "An unfinished business: discrimination in law against persons affected by leprosy and their family members" at the 76th session of the UNGA, bringing attention to the existence of discriminatory laws that still exist throughout the world.[63]

These developments at the UN to follow up on the implementation of the principles and guidelines for the elimination of discrimination against persons affected by leprosy and their families, could not have been achieved without the diligent efforts of Mr. Sasakawa.

4. Conclusion: Aiming for a leprosy-free world

An international leprosy summit, co-organized by the WHO and the Nippon Foundation, called "Overcoming the Remaining Challenges" was held from 24 to 26 July 2013 in Bangkok, Thailand. Ministers from seventeen countries annually reporting over 1,000 cases of leprosy, and relevant stakeholders, including the Nippon Foundation and the WHO, adopted the "Bangkok Declaration: Towards a Leprosy-free World".[64]

Signatories declared that "it is time for the leprosy-endemic countries, as well as their international and national partners, to reaffirm their commitments and reinforce their participation towards addressing leprosy in order to ensure a leprosy-free world at the earliest" (para. 1). Moreover, urging "governments and all interested parties to accord higher priority for activities towards a leprosy-free world, and allocate increased resources in the coming years, in a sustainable manner", the declaration sought to

(a) aim to reduce the burden of leprosy and ultimately move towards a leprosy-free world; (b) apply special focus on high-endemic geographic areas within countries through vigorous and innovative approaches towards timely case detection and treatment completion aiming to achieve leprosy elimination as a public health problem at subnational levels … [and]

(f) promote empowerment of persons affected by leprosy and ensure effective implementation of United Nations resolutions A/RES/65/215, Elimination of Discrimination Against Persons Affected by Leprosy and their Family Members, and A/HRC/RES/15/30 Principles and Guidelines for the Elimination of Discrimination against Persons Affected by Leprosy and their Family Members [para. 2].[65]

At this conference, the Nippon Foundation pledged its intent to provide funds up to a total of US$20 million over the next five years, for the revitalization of activities for countries affected by leprosy.

A "leprosy-free world" means not only the elimination of leprosy as a public health problem, but also the realization of a world free of prejudice or discrimination towards persons affected by leprosy and their family members. Needless to say, we must never repeat the mistakes that were made in the past in many parts of the world, when persons affected by leprosy were discriminated against and isolated. In order for these kinds of tragedies not to be repeated, Mr. Sasakawa is supporting initiatives to preserve the negative history of the forced segregation of persons affected by leprosy, the deprivation of their individual dignity and the various restrictions on their rights that occurred in numerous countries. These preservation efforts include documenting the life histories of persons affected by leprosy, who, despite the harsh lives they were forced to lead and the discrimination they endured, sought to live with strength and dignity, as well as preserving the facilities and leprosaria where they were incarcerated.[66]

Certainly, these kinds of compulsory isolation policies and rights restrictions of persons affected by leprosy are violations of human rights, and must definitely not be models for future generations. However, the past is not something simply to be discarded; it holds the wisdom for a better future. In that sense, we must never forget to learn from the past history of discrimination towards persons affected by leprosy, so that we do not create new forms of discrimination in the future. The "Don't Forget Leprosy" campaign started by Mr. Sasakawa during the COVID-19 pandemic derives from such thinking.

The three pillars of Mr. Sasakawa's work on leprosy are: 1) the medical aspect of eliminating the disease; 2) the social aspect of eliminating the stigma and discrimination against persons affected by leprosy and their family members and restoring their dignity as a human rights issue; and 3) efforts to preserve the history of leprosy, in order to prevent the recurrence of such kinds of cruel prejudice and discrimination and teach us what we need to keep in mind when tackling all kinds of new infectious diseases that we may encounter in the future.

In 2018, the Global Partnership for Zero Leprosy (GPZL) was established through an alliance of international NGOs, support groups and international organs such as ILEP, the Novartis Foundation, the Sasakawa Health Foundation and the World Health Organization. The author looks forward to the results of this new initiative to achieve a leprosy-free world.

2

ELIMINATION OF LEPROSY AS A PUBLIC HEALTH PROBLEM

Derek Lobo

Introduction

The elimination of leprosy as a public health problem globally by the year 2000 and in almost all endemic countries by the year 2010 is one of the most remarkable success stories in the global health sector. It was achieved due to the leadership and direction provided by the World Health Organization (WHO), the effective implementation of multidrug therapy (MDT) and related activities by the endemic countries and the efforts of a large number of leprosy workers at all levels, assisted by technical and financial support from international and national NGOs.

Both the WHO and the national governments of the endemic countries received the highest level of financial, material and moral support from the Nippon Foundation (TNF) and the Sasakawa Memorial Health Foundation (now Sasakawa Health Foundation, or SHF) of Japan, starting from 1975. The founder and initiator of

both TNF and SHF was Mr. Ryoichi Sasakawa, a renowned indus-
trialist and philanthropist from Japan, who had developed an abid-
ing interest in leprosy in his youth and determined that one day he
would make it his business to rid the world of the disease.

By the early 1980s, Mr. Ryoichi Sasakawa handed over the
mantle of responsibility for leprosy elimination to his son, Yohei,
who took on this mission with passion and commitment.

If I have to name a single person who has contributed the most
to the achievement of the goal of elimination of leprosy as a public
health problem, it is Mr. Yohei Sasakawa. For more than forty
years, he has worked relentlessly and steadfastly towards the goal
of a leprosy-free world, and for the past twenty of these (since
2001) he has directed his time, knowledge, experience and efforts
first as the WHO Special Ambassador for the Global Alliance for
the Elimination of Leprosy (2001–2004) and then as WHO
Goodwill Ambassador for Leprosy Elimination (2004 to date). He
has also spearheaded the fight against the stigma and discrimination
associated with leprosy.

The collaboration between the WHO and the Nippon
Foundation started in 1975, when TNF under the leadership of
Mr. Ryoichi Sasakawa contributed US$1.004 million to the WHO
budget for leprosy. WHO's Director-General Dr. Halfdan Mahler
requested that half this amount be used for the smallpox eradication programme, which was short of funds, and Mr. Sasakawa
agreed. The half that went to the leprosy programme enabled the
WHO to provide funding for implementation of critical activities
in high-endemic countries, in addition to advice and recommendations. To quote Dr. H. Sansarricq, then Chief of the WHO Global
Leprosy Unit: "As a consequence of the Sasakawa grant of
US$502,000, government authorities and WHO officials at all
levels—country representatives, regional advisers, and headquarters leprosy staff—grew increasingly confident and enthusiastic
about the feasibility of controlling leprosy at the global level."[1]

The contributions of TNF/SHF to the WHO Leprosy Unit were
in support of a "public health approach" to deal with a communicable disease—leprosy—and for the WHO in turn to support
national leprosy elimination programmes in this approach, with

leprosy services integrated into the general health services. This was a very effective model that from the beginning produced significant results, and it was gradually adopted by other international and national NGOs who had been running their own leprosy asylums, hospitals, clinics and other leprosy services independently, with limited or little collaboration with government.

TNF/SHF and Mr. Ryoichi Sasakawa, and then his son, thus gave a new direction to leprosy work. It was Mr. Yohei Sasakawa who promoted collaboration among all stakeholders. In order to achieve "elimination", he wrote, in the first issue of his ambassador's newsletter in April 2003, "it is necessary to bring together a variety of different actors, such as WHO, the World Bank, national governments, international organizations and NGOs". Mr. Sasakawa was thus able to successfully present a "common goal" to all stakeholders and create a political movement towards elimination.

1. Concept and justification of the goal of elimination of leprosy as a public health problem

The goal of elimination of a communicable disease as a public health problem was first applied by the World Health Organization to leprosy. The initiators and proponents of the concept were Dr. S. K. Noordeen, then Chief of the WHO Global Leprosy Unit, and Dr. Yo Yuasa, Executive and Medical Director of the Sasakawa Health Foundation. The latter had earlier proposed a similar initiative for the WHO's Western Pacific Region.

Key to elimination was the introduction of multidrug therapy (MDT) and the opportunity it provided to make progress against leprosy. Growing antimicrobial resistance to dapsone had led the WHO Scientific Working Group on the Chemotherapy of Leprosy (THELEP), in 1982, to endorse and recommend MDT, a combination of three drugs—rifampicin, clofazimine and dapsone—as an alternative to dapsone monotherapy.

Trials of MDT suggested that if it was implemented vigorously in all endemic countries, it would substantially reduce the leprosy prevalence and burden globally. However, in the absence of a preventive vaccine, and in consideration of a large pool of leprosy cases to be detected in all endemic countries, estimated to be from 10 to 12 million in 1980 to 1985, the WHO decided to propose an "intermediate" goal of eliminating leprosy as a public health problem—with elimination defined as reducing leprosy prevalence to less than one case per 10,000 population—by the year 2000. This was later extended to 2005, when it became apparent that not every country would be able to achieve this target by the year 2000.

In other words, "elimination as a public health problem" meant a reduction in the size of the problem to extremely low levels and not elimination of the disease or eradication—the complete absence of the disease from the community—which was not technically feasible with the tools available and level of knowledge at the time. But it was a clear and achievable goal that leprosy workers at all levels could easily relate to, with a definite target date.

This was the hope and vision of the initiators of the concept, which was adopted at the 44th World Health Assembly in 1991: that it would focus minds and mobilize public health programmes, providing an opportunity made possible by MDT to make hitherto undreamt of advances against leprosy. This was to be achieved, it was hoped, by reducing the number of active cases, leading to a smaller number of sources of infection and eventually leading to a reduction in incidence of the disease.

For Mr. Sasakawa, who was to become the ambassador for leprosy elimination, the setting of a numerical target was very important for motivating health workers and securing political commitment, and was a decision he valued highly.

2. Overview of the leprosy situation prior to availability of MDT

The global leprosy burden from 1980 to 1985, prior to the availability of multidrug therapy (MDT) was as follows:

- There were 122 countries with a national leprosy prevalence of more than one case per 10,000 population, with India topping the list at 58 per 10,000 population and many countries exceeding the figure of 10 per 10,000 population.

- The 122 countries reporting endemic disease (prevalence rate >1 per 10,000 population) together accounted for an estimated global prevalence of 10–12 million cases.[2]
- WHO had recorded approximately 3.6 million cases from 154 countries, with five of these—Brazil, India, Indonesia, Myanmar and Nigeria—accounting for more than 80% of the cases.
- The leprosy programmes in many endemic countries were reporting increasing numbers of dapsone-resistant cases, since dapsone monotherapy was the treatment strategy for leprosy at that point.

In the early 1980s, three positive developments in favour of leprosy control occurred:

(1) In 1981–2, the WHO Study Group on Chemotherapy of Leprosy for Control Programmes recommended the use of multidrug therapy (MDT), a combination of three drugs—rifampicin, clofazimine and dapsone—for treatment of leprosy.
(2) The classification of leprosy for field and treatment purposes was simplified into just two types: (a) paucibacillary (PB) and (b) multibacillary (MB). Two drugs—rifampicin and dapsone—were recommended for PB leprosy and three drugs—rifampicin, clofazimine and dapsone—for MB leprosy.
(3) In view of the potency and efficacy of MDT, the duration of treatment was reduced to 6 months for PB leprosy and 12 months (initially 24 months) for MB leprosy.

3. Challenges of MDT implementation

The implementation of multidrug therapy (MDT) for all detected cases and ensuring treatment completion in six months for PB leprosy and twelve months for MB leprosy, commencing in the mid-1980s in phases and countrywide from the early 1990s in all endemic countries, brought about a dramatic decline in cases worldwide. In addition, it substantially addressed the problem of dapsone resistance.

However, it is one thing to have an effective tool like MDT, but it is a another to provide and deliver the drugs to all endemic countries, and then for the national programmes of endemic countries to effectively implement the leprosy elimination programme countrywide.

Implementation includes many activities such as: case detection, prompt and proper treatment, case holding, completion of treatment within the stipulated duration and ensuring cure, training of staff, creating awareness, ensuring proper treatment and management of complications, disability prevention, Information, Education and Communication (IEC) activities, advocacy, supervision/monitoring, and the logistics involved in transporting, stocking and ensuring delivery of MDT to all those who are diagnosed with leprosy.

This was a challenge that the World Health Organization recognized and met through three key policy initiatives:

1) In May 1991, the World Health Assembly (WHA) passed Resolution 44.9 calling on member countries to aim at "the global elimination of leprosy as a public health problem by the year 2000", defining elimination as reduction of prevalence of leprosy to a level below one case per 10,000 population. The resolution was strongly supported by the Nippon Foundation (TNF) and the Sasakawa Health Foundation, which had been financially supporting the WHO Global Leprosy Unit since 1975.

2) The resolution resulted in increased commitment at the highest political level and enhanced funding by national governments as well as international and national NGOs working for leprosy control in endemic countries. Thereafter, identical resolutions were also adopted at the WHO regional assemblies.

3) As part of the national commitment, most endemic countries appointed a National Task Force (NTF) and a National Steering Committee (NSC), with members drawn from public health specialists, leprologists, scientists, researchers, representatives of leprosy NGOs, and influential opinion builders.

4) The high-level political commitment in turn motivated health administrators at the sub-national levels—state, district and sub-district levels and the peripheral health facilities—who were enthused to carry out vigorous implementation of MDT and related activities like case detection, case holding, supervi-

sion and monitoring, training, IEC, advocacy, awareness creation, etc.

5) Following the 1991 World Health Assembly resolution, the WHO realized that one of the major problems hindering effective MDT implementation was supply and delivery of quality drugs. Dr. S. K. Noordeen, then Chief of the WHO Global Leprosy Unit, discussed this problem with Dr. Yo Yuasa, then Executive and Medical Director of the Sasakawa Health Foundation, and together they presented the problem to the TNF board through Mr. Yohei Sasakawa. Mr. Sasakawa prevailed upon TNF to sponsor the entire MDT drug requirement for five years from 1995 to 1999, with the drugs to be supplied free of charge through the WHO.

6) This example of "drug security" for elimination of a communicable disease was the first of its kind, and also the first model of collaboration between the WHO and an international NGO—the Nippon Foundation. As a ripple effect, the example of TNF sponsorship of MDT was followed by that of pharmaceutical company Novartis, who took over sponsorship of free MDT supply from the year 2000 onwards, an arrangement that continues to this day. The list of endemic countries that received free MDT supply through donation by TNF is given in Appendix 1.

7) In the 1980s, and prior to that, leprosy treatment and care was provided through a specialized vertical structure, in most endemic countries by national governments, along with many international and national NGOs who were dedicated to leprosy work and had established their own asylums, hospitals, leprosy clinics, rehabilitation centres and control programmes. These facilities and services were concentrated mostly on the outskirts of some cities or towns and in some rural areas. They had limited coverage in terms of populations served and patients diagnosed and treated.

8) In view of the above, the WHO strongly advocated the integration of leprosy services into the general health services. The leadership of the vertical programme approach strongly resisted, but the WHO persisted in encouraging national

governments to integrate leprosy services into the general health services. In this, it was supported by TNF and SHF, and also by the World Bank, which came forward to support leprosy elimination activities in countries such as India.

9) Integration resulted in increased geographical and patient coverage of leprosy services, including MDT implementation. For example, in India, MDT treatment was made available in 183,359 government health facilities such as district hospitals, medical college hospitals, community health centres, primary health centres and sub-centres, in addition to the limited number of NGO clinics.

10) Integration also had another important benefit: it reduced the stigma attached to leprosy because now leprosy patients were sitting side-by-side with non-leprosy patients coming for treatment at government health facilities.

Outcome of WHA Resolution, free MDT supply and integration of leprosy services into the general health services

By the end of the year 2000, as a result of the three policies initiated by the WHO, global leprosy prevalence had been reduced to less than one case per 10,000 population, while 108 of the 122 leprosy-endemic countries had attained the goal of elimination of leprosy as a public health problem at the national level. However, some major endemic countries such as Brazil, India, Myanmar, Nepal, Mozambique, Madagascar, Angola, Central African Republic, Democratic Republic of Congo and Tanzania missed the goal, resulting in WHO extending the target date to December 2005.

By 2002, the number of countries reporting endemic leprosy had dropped from 122 to 14. This number subsequently dropped further to 9 countries by 2003. At the end of 2003, these countries—India, Brazil, Nepal, Mozambique, Madagascar, Angola, Central African Republic, Democratic Republic of the Congo and United Republic of Tanzania—accounted for 84% of the global prevalence and 88% of the 515,000 new cases detected. From the 1980s through 2004, more than 14 million cases of leprosy had been treated with MDT.

Excluding small island states with populations under 1 million, the fourteen countries that missed reaching the goal by 2000 were Brazil, India, Indonesia, Myanmar, Nepal, Ethiopia, Madagascar, Mozambique, Angola, Democratic Republic of Congo, Gabon, Ivory Coast, Congo (Brazzaville) and Tanzania. Of the fourteen countries that missed achieving the goal of "Elimination of leprosy as a Public Health Problem" by the year 2000, eight achieved the goal by 2005.

4. Mr. Sasakawa appointed as an Ambassador for Leprosy Elimination

In 1999, when the WHO realized that some countries would not be able to achieve the elimination goal by 2000, it formed the Global Alliance for the Elimination of Leprosy (GAEL) in order to sustain political will and commitment towards implementation of MDT and other leprosy activities, and to give a further boost to the Global Leprosy Programme. In 2001, WHO and GAEL decided to nominate a Special Ambassador to GAEL and the choice was obvious—Mr. Yohei Sasakawa, who had taken up his father Mr. Ryoichi Sasakawa's commitment to a world without leprosy, and was strongly supportive of WHO's initiatives. Subsequently, in 2004, Mr. Sasakawa was appointed as WHO Goodwill Ambassador for Leprosy Elimination.

The appointment of Mr. Sasakawa as the WHO Goodwill Ambassador for Leprosy Elimination started another chapter in Mr. Sasakawa's quest for and commitment to a world without leprosy. He started making more frequent visits to leprosy-endemic countries, particularly those that had not yet achieved the elimination goal by the year 2000, and delivered three key messages wherever he went: Leprosy is curable; Treatment is free; Social discrimination has no place.

The appointment of Mr. Sasakawa as the WHO Special Ambassador on behalf of GAEL had been made in 2001 by Dr. Gro Harlem Brundtland, who was then WHO Director-General. Subsequently, it was Dr. Jong-Wook Lee, who took over as WHO Director-General in 2003, who appointed Mr. Sasakawa as WHO Goodwill Ambassador for Leprosy Elimination.

One of the early decisions taken by Dr. Lee, in consultation with Mr. Sasakawa and his team, was to shift the Global Leprosy Unit from Geneva to the WHO Regional Office for South-East Asia (SEARO) in New Delhi. This was a justifiable and practical move, since the WHO South-East Asia Region accounted for the highest burden of leprosy and included India and Indonesia, the countries reporting the largest and third largest number of cases globally. The WHO's Global Leprosy Programme remains based in New Delhi to this day.

5. Contributions of TNF/SHF to WHO and national programmes

The contributions of TNF/SHF to the WHO Global Leprosy Unit from 1975 to 2021 have exceeded US$200 million. In addition to the US$50 million for the supply of MDT drugs free of charge through WHO from 1995 to 1999, TNF/SHF have contributed to the national leprosy programmes of many endemic countries and to various initiatives to further the cause of leprosy elimination. Needless to say, all these activities have received the backing of Mr. Sasakawa.

(i) Special action projects for the elimination of leprosy (SAPEL)—1995–2002

Special action projects for the elimination of leprosy (SAPELs) were launched in 1995 with the objective of providing MDT services to patients living in difficult-to-access areas or to those belonging to neglected population groups. Difficult-to-access areas are defined as geographically remote places and urban or peri-urban slums where health care infrastructure does not exist or where existing health care services are unable to deliver MDT services. Particular attention was focused on neglected population groups in order to promote equity in health care. This initiative was one of several projects supported by the WHO to help national programmes achieve the goal of eliminating leprosy as a public health problem.

National programmes were encouraged to review the geographical coverage of their MDT services and to identify specific areas and populations where special efforts were needed to reach and treat patients. The WHO actively supported SAPELs in endemic countries by providing technical and financial support to national programmes to implement these projects.

TNF/SHF were the major contributors to the SAPEL initiative. In addition to TNF/SHF, various partners working in endemic countries provided funds, logistic support and human resources.

(ii) Leprosy elimination campaigns (LECs) in support of elimination of leprosy

Leprosy elimination campaigns (LECs) were conducted in highly endemic countries with the aim of improving peripheral-level health services to provide patients with easy access to diagnosis and treatment. The three main objectives of the campaigns are: 1) to build capacity for local health workers; 2) to increase public aware-ness of the disease and involve the community in various leprosy elimination activities; and 3) to diagnose cases that, for various reasons, have remained undetected in the community, and provide free multidrug therapy (MDT) to ensure that patients are cured.

Most endemic countries carried out a single round of LECs. In some countries, like India, LECs were repeated, particularly in areas where routine activities were weak, and to further strengthen the integration of leprosy services and improve community aware-ness. India implemented modified leprosy elimination campaigns (MLECs) in many high-endemic states/districts.

The three objectives of the LECs, initiated in 1995, were adapted by national programmes in the light of local needs and conditions. As a result of capacity-building and awareness-promo-tion activities, a large number of new cases were diagnosed during campaigns and MDT treatment was started promptly.

The LECs were partly or mainly sponsored by TNF/SHF.

(iii) Global Alliance for the Elimination of Leprosy (GAEL)—1999

As mentioned above, the Global Alliance for the Elimination of Leprosy (GAEL) was initiated by the WHO in 1999 when it had become clear that the target set for the elimination of leprosy as a public health problem would not be reached in many high-endemic countries by the year 2000. It was formed at the 3rd International Conference on Elimination of Leprosy at Abidjan, Ivory Coast. At this conference, "The Final Push Strategy to Eliminate Leprosy as a Public Health Problem" was also endorsed.

TNF made a contribution of US$24 million for the activities of GAEL, specifically for "The Final Push Strategy".

(iv) Sponsorship of international conferences, seminars and training programmes

Starting from the 11th International Leprosy Congress, held in Mexico City in 1978, all world leprosy congresses have been partly or mainly supported by TNF/SHF. In addition, many of the seminars, workshops and training programmes related to leprosy, international as well as national, held under the banner of the WHO, have been partially or fully supported by TNF/SHF.

International Leprosy Congresses partly or mainly supported by TNF/SHF:

11th (1978) Mexico City; 12th (1984) New Delhi, India; 13th (1988) The Hague, Netherlands; 14th (1993) Orlando, Florida, USA; 15th (1998) Beijing, China; 16th (2002) Salvador, Brazil; 17th (2008) Hyderabad, India; 18th (2013) Brussels, Belgium; 19th (2016) Beijing, China; 20th (2019) Manila, Philippines; 21st (2022) Hyderbad, India.

(v) Sponsorship of training materials such as Atlas of Leprosy

The Atlas of Leprosy was first published in 1981 and revised in 1983. The aim was to strengthen leprosy control activities by providing high-quality colour pictures as an aid to recognition and early diagnosis of leprosy. It was developed by Dr. Yo Yuasa, Executive and Medical Director of the SHF, in close collaboration with the Leonard Wood Memorial Laboratory in Cebu, the Philippines. The *Atlas* was fully funded by the SHF.

In 2002, *A New Atlas of Leprosy* was published that incorporated some changes in content and format. Almost all the photographs in the original *Atlas* were from the Philippines; these were replaced with photographs of leprosy patients from India and Southeast Asia, where the majority of leprosy cases are found. The 2002 volume was produced by the eminent leprologist Dr. A. Colin McDougall (1924–2006), with additional input from Dr. Yuasa. Once again the printing and distribution of the *Atlas* was fully sponsored by the SHF.

In 2019, *A New Atlas of Leprosy (Revised and Updated)* was published by SHF. It builds on the two previous versions of the *Atlas* and was compiled with technical assistance from the Schieffelin Institute of Health—Research and Leprosy Centre, Karigiri, Tamil Nadu, India, and the WHO's Global Leprosy Programme. This latest *Atlas* brings the contents in line with the WHO Guidelines for the diagnosis, treatment and prevention of leprosy, published in 2018, and also with the WHO's Global Leprosy Strategy 2016–2020, *Accelerating towards a leprosy-free world* and its Operational Manual. The *Atlas* has been endorsed by the Goodwill Ambassador, who describes it as "an excellent reference tool for use in the field" that he hopes "will contribute to the accurate and timely detection of as many new cases as possible".

(vi) Sponsorship of research activities related to leprosy—treatment, vaccines, immunology, pathology, nerve involvement, etc.

The Sasakawa Health Foundation and the Nippon Foundation provided funding to research projects on various aspects of leprosy in a number of countries, in addition to research carried out under the auspices of the WHO Global Leprosy Unit in Geneva.

In 1963, India was the first country to receive a grant from the Nippon Foundation (at that time called the Japan Shipbuilding Industry Foundation) for a leprosy programme. This grant was given through the Tokyo-based voluntary organization the Japan Leprosy Mission to Asia (JALMA) to establish the Central JALMA Institute for Leprosy in Agra. This institute came into existence on

1 April 1976 when the India Centre of JALMA which had been established in 1966 (and managed by JALMA) was officially handed over to the Government of India and subsequently to the Indian Council of Medical Research. The Central JALMA Institute for Leprosy was renamed the "National JALMA Institute of Leprosy and other Mycobacterial Diseases" in 2005 to reflect its broader research areas. The institute is one of the fine examples of international human cooperation and compassion for each other. A sixty-bed hospital with facilities for research and including an electro-static therapy ward, along with electrostatic therapy equipment, a low temperature laboratory and research equipment was opened in 1970.

The two foundations have also supported research in Thailand, the Philippines, South Korea and Malawi. Research fields have included vaccines, drugs, immunology, pathology, nerve involve-ment, "lepra reactions", rehabilitation, social aspects, and stigma and discrimination—in essence, all aspects of leprosy.

(vii) **Sponsorship of the National Forum of People Affec-ted by Leprosy in India (renamed Association of People Affected by Leprosy, or APAL, in 2014), a platform designed to help persons affected make their voices heard and become agents of change.**

6. **Visits of Mr. Sasakawa as WHO Goodwill Ambassador to leprosy-endemic countries as part of leprosy elimination efforts**

In his role as WHO Special Ambassador and WHO Goodwill Ambassador for Leprosy Elimination, Mr. Sasakawa visited over 100 countries between 2001 and 2021. This includes over sixty visits to India—the country with the highest burden of leprosy worldwide.

His schedule usually includes a meeting with the head of state or prime minister, minister of health, senior officials of the Ministry of Health, and programme managers for leprosy elimination at the national and sub-national levels. He also makes a point of meeting and interacting with persons affected by leprosy, particularly those who reside in leprosy self-settled colonies in many countries. He also meets the press to draw attention to leprosy issues and create awareness on the facts of the disease, particularly emphasizing that leprosy is curable, that there is effective treatment and a need to accept and integrate those affected by the disease into the mainstream of society. He also gathers information on leprosy elimination activities in the respective countries and learns about the challenges and problems, so that he can in turn bring them to the attention of policymakers and administrators.

In countries that had achieved the WHO goal of elimination of leprosy as a public health problem by the year 2000, he stressed the need to continue efforts against the disease in order to sustain prevalence below one case per 10,000 population, and to aim at achieving the goal at sub-national levels. He also motivated programme officers to particularly focus on high-endemic pockets and on prevention of disabilities through early case detection and proper management of deformities and disabilities.

In countries that did not achieve the elimination goal by the year 2000, Mr. Sasakawa campaigned for increasing and strengthening activities related to case detection, treatment with MDT, achieving high cure rates, etc., in order to achieve the goal by the year 2005. Thanks to his sustained engagement with national governments, eight out of the fourteen countries that had missed the elimination goal by the year 2000 achieved the goal by the end of 2005. The most prominent country to achieve the goal was India—a spectacular achievement that saw prevalence come down from 58 per 10,000 population in 1980 to less than one case per 10,000 population by the end of 2005 (Maps 1, 2 and 3).

Mr. Sasakawa deserves much credit for this achievement in India because of his frequent advocacy at the highest levels of government at national as well as state levels.

I had the privilege of accompanying Mr. Sasakawa when he visited Bihar, a state highly endemic for leprosy; I also accompanied him once in Indonesia. Hence I have personally witnessed the positive impact of his visits. The very fact that he had an audience with the head of state or the prime minister of a country, or the chief minister of a state or province in large countries, resulted in the

Map 1: Global leprosy situation in 2006: 116 of the 122 leprosy-endemic countries achieved the goal of elimination of leprosy as a public health problem

Leprosy registered prevalence rate per 1,000,000 population: 2006, WHO Global Health Observatory. Geneva: World Health Organization; 2022, (https://apps.who.int/neglected_diseases/ntddata/leprosy/leprosy.html?geog=0&indicator=i0&date=2006&bbox=-230.24

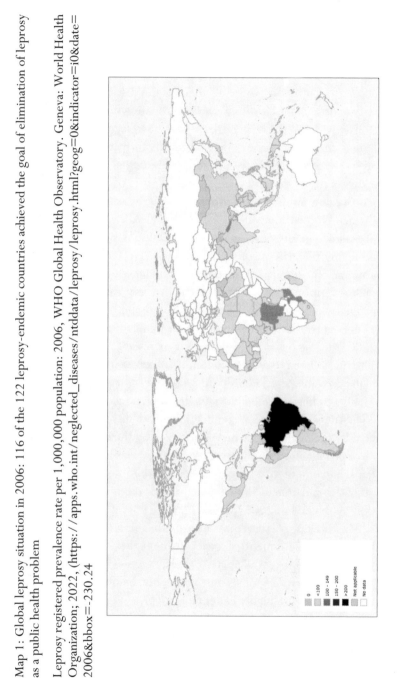

Map 2: Global new leprosy cases, 2006

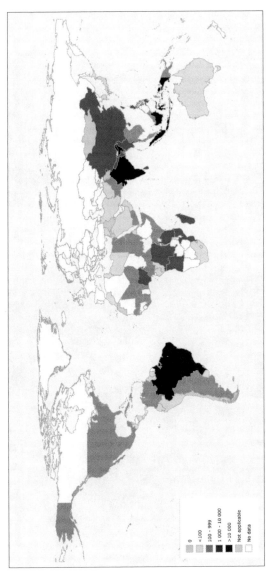

Number of new leprosy cases: 2006, WHO Global Health Observatory. Geneva: World Health Organization; 2022, (https://apps.who.int/neglected_diseases/ntddata/leprosy/leprosy.html?geog=0&indicator=i0&date=2006&bbox=-230.24100000000004,-62.89700000000006,230.24100000000004,90.59700000000002&printmode=true&geog=0&indicator=i0&date=2006&bbox=-230.24100000000004,-92.7596459143969,230.24100000000004,120.4596459143969&printmode=true, accessed 28 March 2023)

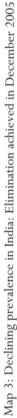

Map 3: Declining prevalence in India: Elimination achieved in December 2005

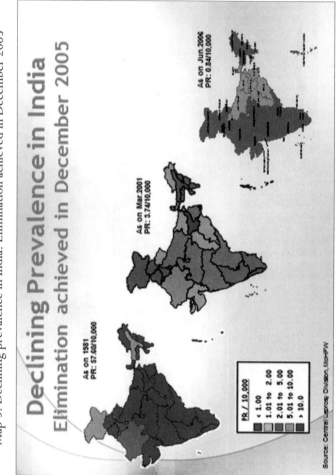

Source: WHO country office, India.

motivation of all administrators at state, province, district and sub-district level to work towards the elimination of leprosy, and encouraged the staff and workers at all levels to vigorously implement leprosy-related activities.

The list of countries visited by Mr. Yohei Sasakawa as WHO Goodwill Ambassador for Leprosy is provided in Appendix 2.

7. Corollary activities related to fighting stigma and discrimination which had an indirect impact on leprosy elimination

(i) The annual Global Appeal to End Stigma and Discrimination against Persons Affected by Leprosy

In his quest for the elimination of leprosy as a disease, as well as his desire to end the related stigma and discrimination, Mr. Sasakawa has, since 2006, organized an annual Global Appeal in collaboration with different partners each year. Though the focus of the Global Appeal is primarily to raise awareness of the issue of stigma and discrimination, the wide publicity that the Global Appeal attracts also highlights the current burden of leprosy and gives momentum to efforts to achieve a world without leprosy.

(ii) WHO Goodwill Ambasssador's Leprosy Bulletin

Since 2003, Mr. Sasakawa has published a bimonthly newsletter in his capacity as WHO Goodwill Ambassador for Leprosy Elimination. The newsletter provides information on leprosy elimination efforts in various countries and also efforts to reduce or prevent stigma, prejudice and discrimination.

The newsletter underwent a redesign and name change in 2020, and now appears as the *WHO Goodwill Ambassador's Leprosy Bulletin*. The publication continues to be an effective organ showcasing the passion and commitment of the Goodwill Ambassador and creating a sense of community by celebrating progress and highlighting challenges at every level of the elimination effort.

(iii) Leprosy—a human rights issue

Deeply concerned about social aspects of the disease, and the stigma and discrimination faced by persons affected by leprosy, including by those who were fully cured, Mr. Sasakawa played a significant role in a successful multi-year effort to gain international recognition for leprosy as a human rights issue through the United Nations. His visit to the Office of the UN High Commissioner for Human Rights (OHCHR) in 2003, and subsequent coordination with the Japanese government, set in motion a process that culminated in 2010 with the UN General Assembly approval of a UN resolution and accompanying principles and guidelines for the elimination of discrimination against persons affected by leprosy and their family members.

(iv) Establishment of the Sasakawa-India Leprosy Foundation (S-ILF)

In 2006, Mr. Sasakawa established the Sasakawa-India Leprosy Foundation (S-ILF), with headquarters in New Delhi, primarily aimed at improving the quality of life and economic well-being of leprosy-affected people in self-settled leprosy colonies in India and their families. There are some 750 such colonies in India and Mr. Sasakawa makes a point of visiting them whenever possible on his trips to that country.

S-ILF supports livelihood programmes, education, scholarships, awareness creation, and the general upkeep of leprosy colonies and economic welfare of the residents of the colonies and their children.

(v) His Holiness Dalai Lama–Sasakawa Scholarships

In 2015, in collaboration with His Holiness the Dalai Lama, Mr. Sasakawa established a scholarship programme for deserving and meritorious youth from the leprosy colonies for higher education and professional qualifications.

A total of 124 youth from leprosy colonies based in nine states of India have so far received the benefit of the scholarships.

Health care and hospitality are two of the most popular courses opted for by the scholars. S-ILF serves as the secretariat of the scholarship programme.

(vi) Establishment of the National Forum of People Affected by Leprosy in India (now known as the Association of People Affected by Leprosy, or APAL)

Post-2005, yet another initiative of Mr. Sasakawa was the formation of the National Forum of People Affected by Leprosy in India to create a platform for people affected to make their voices heard. In 2014, the National Forum changed its name to the Association of People Affected by Leprosy (APAL). He has also supported the activities of organizations of persons affected by leprosy in other countries, including Brazil and Ethiopia.

8. Post-2005—the absence of a clear goal and target date

One of the disappointing factors after 2005, when most countries had achieved the goal of elimination of leprosy as a public health problem at the national level, was the decision of the WHO not to propose a new target but only a vague goal—"to further reduce the burden of leprosy". Considering the significant success of the elimination goal—achieved by 116 of the original 122 leprosy endemic countries by 2005—the WHO's decision was certainly strange and disappointing and, in my personal opinion, unscientific.

It is to the credit of Mr. Sasakawa that he continued his worldwide activities promoting "A world without leprosy" in spite of the absence of a clear goal and target date from the WHO. And it is to the credit of many national governments that they continued to pursue the elimination goal, this time at the sub-national level. The visits of Mr. Sasakawa to those countries helped to sustain political commitment at the highest level and encourage their continued efforts against leprosy in the face of competing priorities. Of the six countries that missed achieving the goal of "Elimination of leprosy as a Public Health Problem" by the year 2005, all but one achieved the goal by 2010.

Map 4: Prevalence rates of leprosy, 2010

Leprosy prevalence rates, data reported to WHO as of beginning January 2010. WHO Global Health Observatory. Geneva: World Health Organization; 2022, (https://www.who.int/images/default-source/maps/leprosy_pr_2009.png?sfvrsn= d5c2c80_0, accessed 28 March 2023)

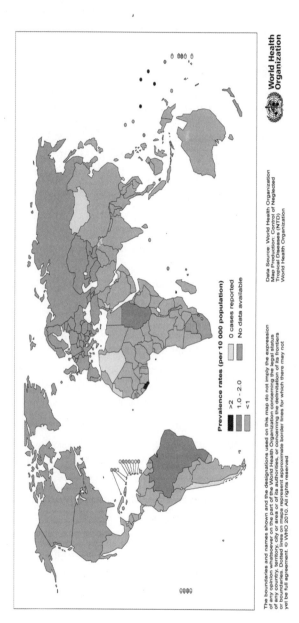

Map 5: Detection rates of new leprosy cases, 2010

Leprosy new case detection rates, data as of beginning January 2010. WHO Global Health Observatory. Geneva: World Health Organization; 2022, (https://www.who.int/images/default-source/maps/leprosy_dr_2009.png?sfvrsn=e613ba44_0, accessed 28 March 2023)

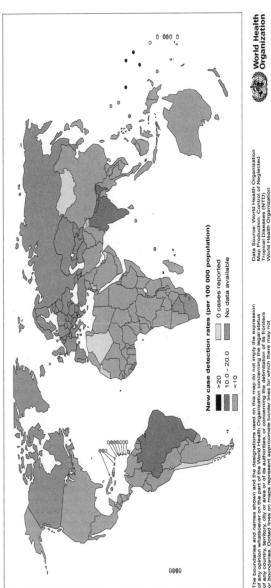

9. "Don't Forget Leprosy" campaign

During the two years from 2020 to 2021, the emergence of COVID-19 has diverted the attention as well as resources of governments and national health programmes towards dealing with the pandemic. This had a negative impact on all communicable and non-communicable disease control programmes and the impact was more pronounced in developing and least-developed countries, where diseases such as leprosy, tuberculosis and other neglected tropical diseases remain endemic.

Mr. Sasakawa was greatly concerned about this situation, and in August 2021 started a campaign called "Don't Forget Leprosy". He wrote to fifty-six health ministers of leprosy-endemic countries and urged them to ensure that the activities related to leprosy were not neglected and every attempt made to see that they continue.

The Sasakawa Health Foundation provided funds for "Don't Forget Leprosy" campaigns in sixteen countries.

10. Conclusion

From 2012 to 2019, the number of newly diagnosed leprosy cases worldwide has held steady at around 200,000. However, since 2015, the number of newly detected cases as well as new cases with Grade-2 disability (G2D) has seen a modest decline each year globally.

Global New Case Detection per Million Population— Steady Decline:

2015 –9.9; **2016** –9.6; **2017** –8.8; **2018** –8.2; **2019** –7.6; **2020** –4.4.

Global New Cases with Grade-2 Disability in Numbers— Steady Decline:

2015 –14,519; **2016** –13,048; **2017** –12,271; **2018** –11,323; **2019** –10,816; **2020** –7,198.

An even more positive and hopeful sign is the fact that in 2020, 31 countries reported zero new leprosy cases; another 31 reported 1–10 new cases; 16 countries reported 11–100 new cases; 34 countries reported 101–1,000 cases; 12 countries reported 1,001–

Table 1: Registered prevalence of leprosy (at end of 2020) and new case detection (during 2020), by WHO Region—WHO Weekly Epidemiological Report, September 2021

WHO Region—*Région OMS*	Number of registered cases at the end of year—*Nombres de cas enregistrés à la fin de l'année*	Prevalence rate (per million population)—*Taux de prévalence (pour 1 million d'habitants)*	Number of new cases detected—*Nombres de nouveaux cas dépistés*	New case detection rate (per million population)—*Taux de dépistage des nouveaux cas (pour 1 million d'habitants)*
Africa—*Afrique*	14,859	13.3	16,690	14.9
Americas—*Amériques*	25,786	25.2	19,195	18.8
Eastern Mediterranean—*Méditerranée orientale*	4,861	6.7	4,077	5.6
European—*Europe*	42	<0.1	27	<0.1
South-East Asia—*Asie du Sud-Est*	78,939	39.1	84,818	42.0
Western Pacific—*Pacific occidental*	4,705	2.4	2,589	1.3
World—*Monde*	**129,192**	**16.6**	**127,396**	**16.4**

[3] World population prospects 2019, online edition revision 1. New York City (NY): United Nations, Department of Economic and Social Affairs, Population Devision: 2019 (http://population.un.org/wpp/ Download/Standard/Population/, accessed July 2021).

[4] Countries are identified as global priorities according to a composite index of parameters such as registered prevalence, new case detection and proportions of female and child cases and of new cases with grade-2 disability (G2D).

[3] *World population prospects 2019, online edition revision 1. New York City (NY): United State, Department of Economic and Social Affairs, Population Division: 2019 (http://population.un.org/wpp/Download/Stardard/Population/, Consulté en Juillet 2021).*

[4] *Les pays prioritaires à l'échelle mondiale sont identifiés sur la base d'un indice composite tenant compte de plusieurs paramètres, dont prévalence enregistrée, les nouveaux cas détectés, la proportion de cas chez la femme et chez l'enfant et la proportion de nouveaux cas présentant une incapacité de degré 2 (ID2).*

10,000 cases; two countries (Brazil and Indonesia) reported 10,000–30,000 cases; and only 1 country—India—reported more than 30,000 cases. Overall, there were 127,396 new cases, a significant decline from the previous year (Table 1).

Even granting that these figures have to be considered in the context of the negative impact of the COVID-19 pandemic on leprosy services, the general situation with regard to leprosy is certainly showing a declining trend. For this, I believe Mr. Yohei Sasakawa deserves credit for the ongoing support and encouragement he has provided to high-endemic countries.

Of course, the real picture will emerge when endemic countries are once again able to fully implement leprosy activities such as case detection and case holding, after the COVID-19 threat subsides. However, we need to take into account the fact that activities such as active case detection throw up respectable numbers of wrong diagnosis or benefit-of-doubt cases or re-registrations. Therefore, the lack of quality and accuracy of diagnosis and a general non-adherence to the WHO-recommended case definitions need to be factored in so as to obtain reliable data on the leprosy situation in each country.

A paper published in 2015 by David J. Blok, Sake J. De Vlas and Jan Hendrick Richardus notes:

> Our projections of future leprosy incidence all show a downward trend. In 2020, the country-level leprosy incidence has decreased to 6.2, 6.1 and 3.3 per 100,000 in India, Brazil and Indonesia respectively, which works out to less than 10 cases per 100,000 population. These three countries account for over 85% of new leprosy cases worldwide. However, elimination is yet to be achieved in some high-endemic regions or high-endemic pockets in all three countries.[3]

In fact, the decline started in 2013 and has continued each year since.

As I mentioned at the outset, the Nippon Foundation and the Sasakawa Health Foundation have been exceptional and unique in providing direct support to the WHO and to national governments in implementing leprosy elimination activities and promoting collective efforts by stakeholders, including international organizations and NGOs.

I can confidently say that the direct support of TNF/SHF to WHO and national programmes was one of the important factors that contributed to the elimination of leprosy as a public health problem globally by the year 2000, and in all leprosy-endemic countries other than Brazil and some small island states by 2010. Therefore, the leaders, policymakers and administrators of TNF/SHF deserve much credit and thanks for their vision, passion, progressive policies and support for the cause of leprosy elimination.

In the meantime, Mr. Sasakawa will have to continue his tireless efforts, utilizing his stature, standing and popularity, and his strong advocacy and public relations capabilities, in order to convince national governments and national leprosy programmes to work towards a leprosy-free world, or zero leprosy, by 2030.

I congratulate Mr. Sasakawa on completion of twenty years of meritorious services as WHO Goodwill Ambassador. He has been a monumental campaigner and advocate for the cause of leprosy elimination—a catalyst, a bridge-builder and a compassionate leader—and I wish, pray and hope that his lifetime dream and vision of "a world without leprosy" will be fulfilled in the near future.

Sources

1. Yohei Sasakawa, *No Matter Where the Journey Takes Me: One Man's Quest for a Leprosy-Free World* (London: Hurst, 2019).
2. Yohei Sasakawa, WHO Goodwill Ambassador for Leprosy Elimination, *My Struggle Against Leprosy* (Tokyo: Festina Lente Japan, 2019).
3. *World Health Organization, Weekly Epidemiological Record* (WER) [on Global Leprosy] 96(36), 10 September 2021, p. 421.
4. Yo Yuasa, *A Life Fighting Leprosy: A Collection of the Speeches and Writings of Dr. Yo Yuasa* [Medical Director—Sasakawa Health Foundation] (Tokyo: Sasakawa Memorial Health Foundation, 2015).
5. Yo Yuasa, *My Family, My Life and My Work: The Autobiography of a Man Who Dreamed of Eliminating Leprosy* (Tokyo: Sasakawa Memorial Health Foundation, 2017).

6. *World Health Organization, MDT Drug Fund 1995–1999 in Collaboration with the Nippon Foundation—Final Report* (World Health Organization, March 2000).

7. Sasakawa Memorial Health Foundation, *Toward a World Without Leprosy—Thirty Years of Sasakawa Memorial Health Foundation* (Tokyo: Sasakawa Memorial Health Foundation, September 2004).

8. Sasakawa-India Leprosy Foundation, *Annual Report 2020–2021*.

Appendix 1: List of endemic countries that received free MDT supply through donation by TNF

No.	Country
1.	Afghanistan
2.	Angola
3.	Argentina
4.	Armenia
5.	Bangladesh
6.	Bolivia
7.	Brazil
8.	Burundi
9.	Cambodia
10.	Cameroon
11.	Central African Republic
12.	China
13.	Colombia
14.	Costa Rica

15.	Cuba
16.	Democratic Republic of Congo
17.	Dominican Republic
18.	Ecuador
19.	Egypt
20.	El Salvador
21.	Equatorial Guinea
22.	Eritrea
23.	Ethiopia
24.	Fiji
25.	Gabon
26.	Ghana
27.	Guatemala
28.	Guinea
29.	Guinea Bissau
30.	Haiti
31.	Honduras
32.	India
33.	Indonesia
34.	Iran
35.	Kazakhstan
36.	Kiribati
37.	Laos

38.	Liberia
39.	Malawi
40.	Maldives
41.	Marshall Islands
42.	Mexico
43.	Micronesia
44.	Mozambique
45.	Myanmar
46.	Nepal
47.	Nicaragua
48.	Nigeria
49.	Northern Mariana Islands
50.	Oman
51.	Pakistan
52.	Panama
53.	Papua New Guinea
54.	Paraguay
55.	Peru
56.	Philippines
57.	Rwanda
58.	Senegal
59.	Sierra Leone
60.	Solomon Islands

61.	Somalia
62.	Sri Lanka
63.	Sudan
64.	Tanzania
65.	Togo
66.	Turkmenistan
67.	Uganda
68.	Uzbekistan
69.	Vanuatu
70.	Venezuela
71.	Vietnam
72.	Western Samoa
73.	Yemen
74.	Zambia
75.	Zimbabwe

Appendix 2: List of countries visited by WHO Goodwill Ambassador for last 20 years

No.	Countries
1.	Angola
2.	Argentina
3.	Azerbaijan
4.	Bangladesh

5.	Belarus
6.	Benin
7.	Bhutan
8.	Brazil
9.	Bulgaria
10.	Burkina Faso
11.	Cambodia
12.	Cameroon
13.	Central African Republic
14.	Chad
15.	Chile
16.	China
17.	Columbia
18.	Comoros Islands
19.	Congo
20.	Costa Rica
21.	Côte d'Ivoire
22.	Cuba
23.	Czech Republic
24.	Democratic Republic of Congo
25.	Ecuador
26.	Egypt

27.	El Salvador
28.	Equatorial Guinea
29.	Ethiopia
30.	Fiji
31.	France
32.	Georgia
33.	Ghana
34.	Honduras
35.	Hungary
36.	Iceland
37.	India
38.	Indonesia
39.	Israel
40.	Italy
41.	Jordan
42.	Kazakhstan
43.	Kenya
44.	Kiribati
45.	Kyrgyzstan
46.	Kenya
47.	Lebanon
48.	Lesotho

49.	Madagascar
50.	Malawi
51.	Malaysia
52.	Mali
53.	Malta
54.	Marshall Islands
55.	Mexico
56.	Micronesia
57.	Montenegro
58.	Morocco
59.	Mozambique
60.	Myanmar
61.	Nepal
62.	Nicaragua
63.	Niger
64.	Nigeria
65.	North Korea
66.	Northern Mariana Islands
67.	Norway
68.	New Zealand
69.	Palau
70.	Peru

71.	Philippines
72.	Papua New Guinea
73.	Portugal
74.	Romania
75.	Russia
76.	Singapore
77.	Slovakia
78.	South Africa
79.	South Korea
80.	Spain
81.	Sri Lanka
82.	Sudan
83.	Sweden
84.	Switzerland
85.	Taiwan
86.	Tajikistan
87.	Tanzania
88.	Thailand
89.	Timor-Leste
90.	Togo
91.	Tunisia
92.	Turkey

A GLOBAL IMPACT

93.	Uganda
94.	Ukraine
95.	United Kingdom
96.	United States of America
97.	Uzbekistan
98.	Vatican City
99.	Vietnam
100.	Zambia

3

LEPROSY AS A HUMAN RIGHTS ISSUE

Takahiro Nanri

Introduction

Leprosy or Hansen's Disease is a chronic infectious disease caused by *Mycobacterium leprae*. It is also called Hansen's disease after Dr. Gerhard Henrik Armauer Hansen, the Norwegian physician who identified the bacillus in 1873. In the past, leprosy was considered an incurable disease, but today it is treatable with multidrug therapy (MDT).

Since leprosy is a disease of low infectiousness, and most people are naturally immune, the risk of getting the disease is very low. However, if a person does contract leprosy, and treatment is delayed, the disease can damage the peripheral nerves, resulting in numbness and motor function loss, and be progressively disfiguring.

Leprosy is one of the oldest diseases in human history. References to a disease thought to be leprosy appear in the Old Testament of the Bible, when the disease was viewed as a divine punishment or a curse and sufferers ostracized.

In the latter half of the nineteenth century, following Hansen's discovery that leprosy was an infectious disease, policies to segregate patients were adopted all over the world, and these were not reconsidered until the second half of the 1950s. Accordingly, even today many people mistakenly believe that leprosy is a highly transmissible, frightening disease, and persons affected by leprosy and their family members face severe discrimination.

In 1948, the United Nations (UN) adopted the Universal Declaration of Human Rights. The first article states: "All human beings are born free and equal in dignity and rights. They are endowed with reason and conscience and should act towards one another in a spirit of brotherhood."[1] However, discrimination towards persons affected by leprosy and their family members transcends political, religious and cultural differences and is found throughout the world. Meanwhile, it is only relatively recently that there has been international recognition of leprosy as a human rights issue, and it was only in 2008 that the United Nations Human Rights Council (UNHRC) first adopted a resolution on Elimination of Discrimination Against Persons Affected by Leprosy and Their Family Members. This resolution was also unanimously approved at the UN General Assembly (UNGA) in 2010, in conjunction with Principles and Guidelines on the Elimination of Discrimination Against Persons Affected by Leprosy and Their Family Members (P&G), indicating the direction that national governments should take in regard to this issue. Subsequently, in November 2017, a UN Special Rapporteur on the Elimination of Discrimination Against Persons Affected by Leprosy and Their Family Members was appointed, and the Special Rapporteur has conducted periodic surveys into different aspects of leprosy and human rights and issued reports.

Playing a central role in the process of mobilizing the international community and establishing the view that leprosy is a human rights issue was Mr. Yohei Sasakawa, the current chairman of the Nippon Foundation and concurrently the World Health Organization (WHO) Goodwill Ambassador for Leprosy Elimination, who also serves as the government of Japan's Goodwill Ambassador for the Human Rights of Persons Affected by Leprosy. Mr. Sasakawa promoted a series of activities in alliance with the Nippon Foundation and the Sasakawa Health Foundation, which had been established to promote scientifically based solutions to leprosy and assist countries in their efforts to tackle the disease.[2] Furthermore, Mr. Sasakawa's efforts to establish the human rights of persons affected by leprosy, a socially vulnerable group who, it is no exaggeration to say, languish at the bottom of society, have a relevance beyond leprosy in that they relate to efforts to address discrimination and improve the human rights situation concerning other illnesses and infectious diseases, and with the commitment embodied in the Sustainable Development Goals (SDGs) to "leave no one behind".

Accordingly, this chapter highlights the background to these activities and the steps taken by Mr. Sasakawa, in collaboration with diverse stakeholders such as organizations of persons affected by leprosy, NGOs, experts and the media, in order to encourage the UN and governments to act. The author also analyzes the kinds of ripple effects brought about by these activities towards the realization of a world without leprosy, that is, a world in which no one suffers from having experienced leprosy. In addition, the author also considers what kind of pointers these activities offer for addressing broader issues of common concern, such as the achievement of the SDGs.

1. Leprosy is a human rights issue

Mr. Sasakawa has said the following about how he came to focus on leprosy as a human rights issue:

> From the time I was appointed as the Special Ambassador of the Global Alliance for the Elimination of Leprosy (GAEL) in 2001,[3] I have visited many countries to realize the elimination of leprosy as a public health issue, or to provide MDT to as many patients as possible. I have gone into the field numerous times, and directly met with many thousands of persons affected by leprosy. As a result, I came to see that, even when treatment for leprosy is completed, it's not the end of the story. In other words, leprosy causes many people to lose their jobs and families, and be excluded from society. Further, I witnessed numerous people who, unable to

return to their former lives, suffered from discrimination and prejudice from society for the rest of their lives. At that time, I belatedly realized that if we did not resolve leprosy as a human rights issue, we would not have truly conquered leprosy.[4]

In October 2001, not long after being appointed GAEL Special Ambassador, Mr. Sasakawa gave the keynote speech at the 5th Forum 2000 conference in Prague, Czech Republic.[5] He spoke on the issue of leprosy and human rights, saying:

> Although we are close to the elimination of leprosy as a medical issue, human rights issues remain deeply rooted. Society has been unaware of this for a very long time. However, whenever we are discussing human rights, we should also consider the major proposition of how we can remove the prejudice towards these people who are in a weak position in society, and have them accepted by society.[6]

At a time when the world was tackling the elimination of leprosy as a public health problem under the leadership of the WHO, it is a testament to Mr. Sasakawa's foresight that he was already talking about leprosy in terms of human rights.[7]

2. Adoption of the Resolution on Elimination of Discrimination Against Persons Affected by Leprosy and Their Family Members by the UN General Assembly

2–1. Approach to the UN Human Rights Commission (2003–2005)

Mr. Sasakawa began in earnest to address leprosy and human rights issues as a result of his meeting in July 2003 with Dr. Bertrand Ramcharan, the UN Acting High Commissioner for Human Rights (OHCHR). At this meeting, Mr. Ramcharan recommended that Mr. Sasakawa hold a side event related to leprosy at the 55th session of the UN Sub-Commission on the Promotion and Protection of Human Rights planned for the following month, as well as arrange a meeting with the UN Special Rapporteur on the Right of Everyone to the Enjoyment of the Highest Attainable Standard of Physical and Mental Health. Following this advice, during the session of the Sub-Commission in August 2003, the Nippon Foundation organized the first ever side event on the topic of leprosy and human rights. Persons affected by leprosy from the US, the Philippines, Ethiopia and India served as panellists, and told of their experiences of human rights violations.

But there was little interest, and only about ten people attended. Shortly thereafter, Mr. Sasakawa held a meeting with Professor Paul Hunt, the UN "Right to Health" Special Rapporteur, then a professor at the University of Essex in England. Professor Hunt showed a certain understanding of leprosy issues, and suggested that there was a possibility that these issues could be addressed within his own mandate as Special Rapporteur.

However, Mr. Sasakawa felt there was a danger that if leprosy was treated the same way as other health concerns, the specific issues would be buried. He decided that leprosy should be taken up independently and to contact the UN Commission on Human Rights directly. At its 60th plenary session held in March 2004, Mr. Sasakawa gave his first oral statement on "leprosy and human rights". Concerning why leprosy had not up until then been treated as a human rights issue, Mr. Sasakawa claimed that "This is because these are abandoned people. They have had both their names and their identity stripped away. They cannot cry out for their rights. They are silenced people."

Subsequently, Mr. Sasakawa took a series of steps to gain the support of the Commission on Human Rights. In May of the same year, he held a briefing on leprosy for staff of the Office of the UN Commission on Human Rights (OHCHR), and during the 56th session of the UN Sub-Commission on the Promotion and Protection of Human Rights in July, he organized a lunch for the Sub-Commission members, with twenty-two out of twenty-six members attending. As a result of all these measures, the Sub-Commission went so far as to pass a resolution entrusting Professor Yozo Yokota, a committee member and at the time a professor at Chuo University in Tokyo, to conduct a study on "discrimination against leprosy-affected persons and their families" and to submit a preliminary survey report to the Sub-Commission the following year.

Thereafter, Mr. Sasakawa met Ms. Louise Arbour, the UN High Commissioner for Human Rights who had been appointed in November of that year, in Tokyo, and made the case for leprosy to be addressed as a human rights issue. As well as receiving Ms. Arbour's agreement, Mr. Sasakawa also actively supported the field surveys and data-collection activities of Professor Yokota in leprosy-endemic countries.

Professor Yokota submitted a report on the results of his surveys at the 57th session of the UN Sub-Commission on the Promotion and Protection of Human Rights held in August 2005. The Sub-Commission adopted a resolution to promote the elimination of leprosy-related discrimination, and appointed the professor as a Special Rapporteur. He was commissioned to undertake further surveys and to submit a report.[8] The resolution largely overlapped with subsequent Human Rights Council resolutions and the P&G, with the Sub-Commission requesting or encouraging governments to prohibit discrimination against persons affected by leprosy and their families; abolish legislation requiring the forced hospitalization of leprosy patients; provide appropriate remedies for those who were forcibly hospitalized; and include education about leprosy in school curricula.[9]

At this session of the UN Sub-Commission on the Promotion and Protection of Human Rights Mr. Sasakawa gave a further oral statement. But he spoke only briefly before giving the floor to persons affected by leprosy from India, Nepal and Ghana, although this had not been part of the original plan.

This was the first opportunity that persons affected by leprosy had ever had to address the Sub-Commission. A year later, in August 2006, Professor Yokota submitted a report to the 58th session of the Sub-Commission on his survey into the actual conditions of discrimination in various countries, with the Sub-Commission endorsing its recommendations.

During this period, Mr. Sasakawa expressed his views through the world's media, submitting articles to major news organizations in various countries, issuing press releases and holding press conferences in conjunction with international conferences and projects organized by the Nippon Foundation, and hosting seminars for representatives of the media.

An example is the article Mr. Sasakawa wrote titled "Conquering an ancient scourge: Leprosy is not a stigma anymore" that appeared in the 18–19 September 2004 weekend edition of the *International Herald Tribune* (published by the New York Times). The fact that an article focusing on leprosy as a human rights issue was featured in a major Western newspaper gave a boost to Mr. Sasakawa's efforts to lobby the Human Rights Commission. However, as part of the structural reform of the UN, the Commission was dissolved after holding its final session in March 2006, followed by the dissolution of the Sub-Commission in August 2006 at the conclusion of its 58th session. Although it appeared that all of Mr. Sasakawa's approaches to the UN Commission on Human Rights had come to naught, Mr. Sasakawa did not give up, but switched his focus to the UN Human Rights Council that replaced it in March 2006.[10]

2–2. Approaches to the UN Human Rights Council (2006–2010)

First, Mr. Sasakawa approached the government of Japan. As a result, at the 2nd session of the UN Human Rights Council in September 2006, the government of Japan issued a statement calling for a follow-up to the resolution on elimination of discrimination against persons affected by leprosy that had been adopted by the Sub-Commission on the Promotion and Protection of Human Rights. Further, Mr. Sasakawa himself sent a document to every member country of the Human Rights Council requesting that they respect the resolution adopted by the Sub-Commission.

In 2007, Mr. Sasakawa was appointed by the government of Japan as its Goodwill Ambassador for the Human Rights of Persons Affected by Leprosy, and during the 6th session of the UN Human Rights Council in the same year, he submitted a written request on leprosy and human rights and also held side events and receptions. Subsequently, Mr. Sasakawa began to work in earnest for a new resolution on elimination of discrimination to be adopted by the Human Rights Council, which was more difficult to attempt. For it should be noted here that resolutions of the Human Rights Council carry greater weight than those adopted by the UN Sub-Commission on the Promotion and Protection of Human Rights, because they are submitted and adopted by member countries.

With the government of Japan agreeing to submit a new draft resolution in response to his approach, Mr. Sasakawa travelled to Geneva in May 2008 and began moves to drum up support for the resolution, visiting the Permanent Missions to the UN of twenty-seven countries. Included among these were countries such as Cuba and China, that normally do not welcome initiatives from the government of Japan. He continued these activities during the 8th session of the Human Rights Council held that June. In the end, the Human Rights Council unanimously adopted a resolution co-sponsored by fifty-nine countries on elimination of discrimination against persons affected by leprosy and their family members (A/HRC/RES/8/13).[11] Exceptionally, as a result of Mr. Sasakawa's efforts, Cuba and China were among the co-sponsors.

The resolution, which recognized that leprosy is not only a medical or health issue but also one of human rights, contained a number of provisions, including: calling on governments to take measures to eliminate discrimination; requesting the OHCHR to include discrimination against persons affected by leprosy as an important matter in its human rights education and awareness-raising activities; requesting the OHCHR to gather information and hold a meeting among relevant actors and transmit a report to the Human Rights Council Advisory Committee; and requesting the Advisory Committee (the successor to the Sub-Commission on the Promotion and Protection of Human Rights) to submit to the Council by September 2009 a draft set of Principles and Guidelines for the Elimination of Discrimination Against Persons Affected by Leprosy and Their Family Members (P&G).

Further, at the 1st session of the Human Rights Council Advisory Committee held in August of the same year, Professor Shigeki Sakamoto, who at the time was a professor at Kobe University, was put in charge of developing the draft Principles and Guidelines. Mr. Sasakawa, as he had done for Professor Yokota, fully supported Professor Sakamoto in his activities to gather data and conduct surveys for the purpose of compiling the P&G.

In accordance with the resolution, on 15 January 2009 the OHCHR held an official consultation at the UN's European headquarters in Geneva, bringing together approximately eighty people comprising representatives of national governments, persons affected by leprosy, international organizations, NGOs and human rights experts. It was the first ever official meeting on leprosy and human rights held at the UN.

The following day, the Nippon Foundation held an informal consultation to allow more time for the voices of stakeholders, especially persons affected by leprosy, to be heard and reflected in the process of compiling the P&G. Concerning the importance of these two consultations, Mr. Sasakawa wrote:

> On the issue of leprosy and human rights, I was concerned that it would be positioned as a so-called "the right to health" issue, that is, the right of all human beings to have equal access to health care and lead healthy lives. Needless to say, there is a need to create the conditions where people can receive diagnoses and appropriate treatment anywhere in the world. However, as far as I know, leprosy is the only disease where discrimination occurs even after the illness is cured. The disease causes a social label to be attached, creating barriers to all aspects of daily life, including education, employment and marriage. These are human rights issues that go far beyond the scope of health. With regard to leprosy and human rights, I see an important distinction between leprosy being positioned as part of health, or separately as a violation of human rights. In the end, "leprosy and human rights" was treated as a separate issue, as I had hoped. [12]

In other words, after the UN Human Rights Council adopted a resolution on elimination of discrimination against persons affected by leprosy and their family members for the first time, it was agreed on at these consultations that leprosy and human rights would be treated as an independent issue. This would greatly boost Mr. Sasakawa's efforts to build up a groundswell of support for leprosy to be framed in a human rights context.

After the Advisory Committee submitted the draft set of principles and guidelines formulated by Professor Sakamoto to the 12th session of the Human Rights Council, the Council adopted a resolution requesting the OHCHR to collect the views of relevant actors, such as governments, UN bodies, NGOs and persons affected by leprosy, and share these views with the Advisory

Committee. It further requested that the Advisory Committee submit a final draft to the Council by its 15th session (A/HRC/RES/12/7).[13]

Then, when the final draft of the P&G was approved at the 15th session of the Human Rights Council held in September 2009, the Council requested a wide range of stakeholders in various countries (from hospitals, schools, universities, business sectors, the media, NGOs, etc.) in addition to national governments, UN organs and human rights bodies, to respect the P&G, and, at the same time, adopted a resolution recommending that the UNGA should adopt the resolution on elimination of discrimination against persons affected by leprosy and their family members (A/HRC/RES/15/10).[14]

Following this recommendation, at the 65th session of the UNGA in December 2010, the resolution and accompanying P&G were adopted unanimously by 193 countries.

2–3. The Principles and Guidelines for the Elimination of Stigma and Discrimination Against Persons Affected by Leprosy and their Family Members

The P&G, which are a road map to eliminate leprosy-related stigma and discrimination, consist of two parts: "principles" and "guidelines" (see Table 2).[15]

First, the "principles" state that persons affected by leprosy and their family members should be treated as people with dignity and are entitled, on an equal basis with others, to all the human rights and fundamental freedoms proclaimed in the Universal Declaration of Human Rights as well as other international human rights instruments. Also, that persons affected by leprosy and their family members should not be discriminated against on the grounds of having or having had leprosy; should have the same rights as others with respect to marriage, family and parenthood; should have the same rights as everyone else in relation to full citizenship and obtaining identity documents; should have the right to serve the public, stand in elections and hold office; should have the right to work; should not be denied admission to or expelled from schools and training programmes on the grounds of leprosy; are entitled to develop their human potential and fully realize their dignity and self-worth; and have the right to participate in decision-making processes regarding policies and programmes that directly concern their lives.

Moreover, the "guidelines" suggest actions for national governments to take in the following fourteen categories: general (full realization of human rights); equality and non-discrimination; women, children and other vulnerable groups; home and family; living in the community and housing; participation in political life; occupation; education; discriminatory language; participation in public cultural and recreational activities; health care; standard of living; awareness-raising; and development, implementation and follow-up to states' activities.

Table 2: Outline of the P&G

Principles
Persons affected by leprosy and their family members are entitled to all the human rights and fundamental freedoms proclaimed in the Universal Declaration of Human Rights and other relevant international human rights instruments.
Guidelines
1. Promote, protect, and ensure the full realization of all human rights and fundamental freedoms for all persons affected by leprosy and their family members.
2. Recognize that all persons are equal before the law and entitled to equal protection of the law.
3. Pay special attention to the promotion and protection of the human rights of women, children and members of other vulnerable groups.
4. Support the reunification of families separated in the past as a result of policies and practices relating to persons diagnosed with leprosy.

5. Promote enjoyment of rights, including choice of place of residence, allowing full inclusion and participation in the community.

6. Ensure rights related to participation in political life.

7. Encourage and support employment.

8. Promote equal access to education.

9. Remove discriminatory language from governmental publications.

10. Promote equal access to public places, public transport, cultural and recreational facilities, and places of worship.

11. Provide free or affordable health care that includes early detection, prompt treatment, counselling, and access to free medication.

12. Recognize the right to an adequate standard of living and provide assistance to persons living in poverty.

13. Raise awareness and foster respect for human rights and dignity.

14. Create a committee of stakeholders to develop, implement, and follow up on activities relating to human rights.

(Source: "Quick Reference Guide: Principles and Guidelines", *WHO Goodwill Ambassador's Leprosy Bulletin*, no. 105, September 2021, p. 7; published by Sasakawa Health Foundation).

3. Appointment of UN Special Rapporteur (2011–2017)

3–1. Establishment of International Working Group (IWG)

For people involved with leprosy issues, the adoption by the UNGA of the resolution and the P&G supported Mr. Sasakawa's view that the fight against leprosy can be compared to the two wheels of a motorcycle, namely, that "the front wheel represents medical treatment with MDT, and the back wheel activities to end stigma and discrimination. And … unless the two wheels turn smoothly at the same speed, there can be no arrival at the 'destination'." That destination, in Mr Sasakawa's words, is the realization of a world without leprosy and without the stigma and discrimination that accompany the illness.[16]

Professor Sakamoto, who oversaw the drafting of the P&G, said the following about their significance: "First, international standards for the human rights of persons affected by leprosy have been established. Second, it has been made clear that persons affected by leprosy are subjects who enjoy human rights under international law."[17]

However, since states were not required to comply with the P&G, a major challenge was how they would be implemented, and whether and how their adoption would in fact lead to the elimination of discrimination in relation to leprosy. As Professor Yokota, who served as the Special Rapporteur for the UN Sub-Commission on the Promotion and Protection of Human Rights, said:

> There were great benefits gained from the fact that the UNGA adopted the resolution for the elimination of leprosy discrimination, and called for respect of the P&G that had been compiled by the Human Rights Council. However, unless the P&G are actually understood by national governments, UN organs, and furthermore non-state bodies such as corporations and other groups, leprosy-related discrimination will not disappear. In that sense, after the adoption of the resolution by the UNGA, it will be important to conduct follow-ups on the actual conditions of implementation by relevant organs and groups.[18]

The adoption by the UNGA of the resolution on elimination of discrimination against persons affected by leprosy and their family members, which duly notes the Principles and Guidelines prepared by the Human Rights Council, was a major achievement, but discrimination will not disappear unless the P&G are understood and implemented by governments, UN bodies and non-state actors such as NGOs, the business sector and other organizations. In that sense, it will be important to follow up on the implementation status in countries and organizations in the wake of the resolution.

In fact, even after this, Mr. Sasakawa continued to focus his energy on promoting the dissemination and implementation of the P&G. With that in mind, he arranged for five symposiums on leprosy and human rights to be held in different parts of the world between 2012 and 2015: Rio de Janeiro, Brazil (January 2012); New Delhi, India (October 2012); Addis Ababa, Ethiopia (September 2013); Rabat, Morocco (November 2014); and Geneva, Switzerland (June 2015).

Following the first symposium in Brazil in 2012, an International Working Group (IWG) on leprosy and human rights comprising thirteen human rights experts from various countries was established, and surveys were begun on the ways that the P&G should be implemented appropriately. Composed of human rights practitioners, researchers, and representatives of groups of persons affected by leprosy, the IWG's members came from Japan, Kuwait, Brazil, the US, the Philippines, Sri Lanka, India, Ethiopia, Jordan and Bulgaria.

The IWG held regular meetings in conjunction with the four international symposiums that followed the initial one in Rio, and in June 2015 released its final report.[19] In the report, as well as suggesting model action plans for appropriately implementing the P&G in each country, the IWG suggested that the UN Human Rights Council recommend to the Human Rights Council Advisory Committee that survey and research on constructing a follow-up mechanism for the appropriate implementation of the P&G should be carried out. This suggestion led to the adoption of a new Human Rights Council resolution that will be discussed below.

3–2. Further approaches to the Human Rights Council

Over the course of the symposiums, and while the IWG carried out surveys, Mr. Sasakawa came to believe that a new Human Rights Council resolution was needed if the P&G were to be properly implemented, as well as further surveys. To start with, he felt it was important to build up a collaborative environment within the Human Rights Council Advisory Committee, and he set up an opportunity to ask directly for the committee's cooperation.

Specifically, during the session of the Advisory Committee in February 2015, he invited all the committee members to a luncheon co-hosted with the Permanent Mission of Japan to the International Organizations in Geneva. Fifteen of the eighteen committee members attended the luncheon, to which representatives of a group of persons affected by leprosy from India and Professor Sakamoto, who had developed the P&G, were also invited.

The participation of persons affected by leprosy and of Professor Sakamoto likely contributed to deepening the committee members' understanding of the issues, because after the luncheon meeting, a number of committee members expressed their intention to cooperate.

Meanwhile, based on what was discussed at the five international symposiums and at meetings of the IWG, Mr. Sasakawa made the case to the Japanese government for a new resolution and succeeded in gaining its support. Further, since the government of Japan needed to get more co-sponsors in order to submit the resolution, the Permanent Mission of Japan to the International Organizations in Geneva worked together with the Nippon Foundation in approaching various countries' diplomatic representatives.

The extensive networks of the Nippon Foundation, which carries out projects in many parts of the world, were fully utilized. Mr. Sasakawa approached the governments of relevant countries in Asia, Europe, Latin America and Africa either directly or indirectly to encourage them to support the resolution. As a result, the resolution was co-sponsored by ninety-seven countries, more than the previous resolution, and was adopted unanimously in July 2015 (A/HRC/RES/29/5).[20]

The five international symposiums held between 2012 and 2015, and the lunch arranged for members of the Human Rights Council Advisory Committee in February 2015, all took place in cooperation with organizations of persons affected by leprosy.

Moreover, in June 2015, during the 29th session of the Human Rights Council, the Nippon Foundation and the Permanent Mission of Japan to the International Organizations in Geneva hosted a side event at the UN Secretariat in Geneva. In addition to an exhibition of photographs, a ceremony was held promoting the importance of leprosy as a human rights issue, with the cooperation of persons affected by leprosy from India, Colombia, Indonesia, Ghana and Morocco.

Mr. Sasakawa's close collaboration with organizations of persons affected by leprosy around the world through the Nippon Foundation was a major driving force in gaining support from the relevant authorities concerning the need for a new resolution on the issue of leprosy and human rights.

3–3. Follow-up on the P&G

The resolution that was adopted by the Human Rights Council in July 2015 requested that the Advisory Committee undertake a survey reviewing the implementation of the P&G and obstacles thereto, and submit a report containing practical suggestions for the wider dissemination and more effective implementation of the P&G to the 35th session of the Human Rights Council in June 2017. This was in accordance with the recommendations of the IWG.

The Advisory Committee duly established a drafting group composed of seven members to prepare the report, with committee member Professor Kaoru Obata of Nagoya University as committee chair, and Mr. Imeru Tamrat Yigezu of Ethiopia as the Rapporteur. Mr. Yigezu conducted surveys on the degree to which there is awareness of the P&G; whether or not there have been specific responses by governments [to discrimination]; the use of discriminatory language; the level of participation by persons affected by leprosy in decision-making processes; challenges faced in regard to the implementation of the P&G; the specific nature of existing discrimination; and other matters.

Through the Nippon Foundation, Mr. Sasakawa supported the collection of data and surveys and the research activities of Mr. Yigezu, which revealed that persons affected by leprosy and their family members continue to face the kinds of discrimination outlined below.[21]

(i) Discrimination against persons affected by leprosy

In India, for example, some persons affected by leprosy live in isolated colonies, among whom some rely on begging to make a living.[22] Moreover, in states such as Rajasthan, Andhra Pradesh, Chhattisgarh and Madhya Pradesh, persons affected by leprosy are not allowed to stand for election. There was also a case in Uttar Pradesh where a group of persons affected by leprosy wanted to hold a conference at a hotel, but were refused.

Furthermore, although persons affected by leprosy nominally have the right to vote, if they live in a colony without owning the land they live on and without residency rights, they are unable to obtain a state-issued identity card, making it impossible for them to exercise their right to vote.

Similar cases were noted in Bangladesh, Myanmar, Vietnam and elsewhere. In Brazil, it was reported that an electoral office refused to issue an election card to a person affected by leprosy on the grounds that the person was illiterate and could not be fingerprinted because of a disability.

In the Democratic Republic of the Congo, it was reported that persons affected by leprosy did not have the right to marry or use the same water to shower as other people because there was still a perception that leprosy was an easily transmissible, incurable disease.

There were also reports of cases in India and Indonesia where persons affected by leprosy were not allowed to receive diagnoses at general hospitals. Although more than five years had elapsed since the UNGA adopted the P&G, Mr. Yigezu's survey showed that the P&G were not sufficiently understood or being properly implemented, and it was clear that deep-rooted discrimination towards persons affected by leprosy and their family members still existed.

(ii) Recommendation of the appointment of a Special Rapporteur

In the last report submitted to the Advisory Committee in February 2017, Mr. Yigezu wrote: "It is therefore highly recommended that a special procedure mandate under the auspices of the Human Rights Council be created for the purpose of following up, monitoring and reporting on progress made and measures taken by States for the effective implementation of the Principles and Guidelines."[23]

In response to this recommendation, Mr. Sasakawa judged that the appointment of a Special Rapporteur on leprosy would be key to the appropriate implementation of the P&G, and secured the government of Japan's support that it would submit a new resolution. At first, some countries were reluctant to adopt the resolution because the establishment of a Special Rapporteur would give rise to new costs; however, the government of Japan (Ministry of Foreign Affairs) actively lobbied the relevant countries.

Mr. Sasakawa himself gave an oral statement to the Human Rights Council, in which he spoke of the necessity of establishing a Special Rapporteur. He also had meetings with government representatives from Brazil and Ethiopia, seeking support for the draft resolution. As a result, at the 35th session of the Human Rights Council in June 2017, a new resolution based on the above report recommending the appointment of a Special Rapporteur on the elimination of discrimination against persons affected by leprosy and their family members (with a term of three years) was adopted (A/HRC/RES/35/9).[24] The resolution, as well as stating the obligation for the Special Rapporteur to report annually to the Human Rights Council, also encouraged the OHCHR and the Special Rapporteur to hold seminars on leprosy-related discrimination in order to widely disseminate the principles and guidelines.

Then, at the Human Rights Council session in November of the same year, Portugal-born Ms. Alice Cruz was appointed as the Special Rapporteur. Three years later, at the 44th session of the Human Rights Council held in June 2020, with the proactive support of Mr. Sasakawa, Ms. Cruz's term as Special Rapporteur was extended for a further three years (A/HRC/RES/44/6).[25]

4. The activities of the Special Rapporteur towards the elimination of leprosy-related discrimination (2017–)

4–1. Appointment of the Special Rapporteur

Mr. Sasakawa expressed his hopes for the Special Rapporteur thus: "With the appointment of the Special Rapporteur, I would like to see her thoroughly investigate the realities of discrimination in each country and, based on the results, urge governments to strictly adhere to the P&G."[26]

Ms. Cruz, the Special Rapporteur, makes country visits, gathers data on discrimination experienced on an everyday level by persons affected by leprosy and their family members, and compiles an annual report for the Human Rights Council session held each year in June.

Mr. Sasakawa, in collaboration with the Nippon Foundation and the Sasakawa Health Foundation, has provided wide-ranging support so that the Special Rapporteur's activities would be more effective. One example of this support was to act as a bridge between the Special Rapporteur and organizations of persons affected by leprosy in different part of the world. As detailed in another chapter, the Nippon Foundation and the Sasakawa Health Foundation have consistently supported the empowerment of persons affected by leprosy for the past quarter of a century, with both foundations establishing close relationships with organizations of persons affected worldwide.[27]

In September 2019, the two foundations co-hosted a conference of people's organizations on Hansen's disease in Manila, the Philippines, in which more than eighty representatives of leprosy-related groups from eighteen countries took part. Ms. Cruz participated in this conference and had the opportunity to converse directly with many affected persons.

In January 2021, the Sasakawa Health Foundation hosted a webinar titled "Zero Leprosy for Whom in the Post-COVID World?", in which representatives of twenty-two leprosy-related groups from seventeen countries participated and discussed the challenges they faced amid the coronavirus pandemic. Ms. Cruz took part in the webinar as a moderator.

Since the number of NGOs and experts tackling leprosy issues is by no means large, a major challenge for Ms. Cruz has been obtaining information from the field. The coronavirus pandemic has exacerbated the difficulties by effectively closing the way to official visits by the Special Rapporteur.

As shown below, since 2018, Ms. Cruz has been submitting a yearly thematic report on leprosy and human rights to the Human Rights Council sessions held every year in June.

4–2. The Annual Reports of the Special Rapporteur

(i) The 2018 Thematic Report

In the 2018 thematic report,[28] which Mr. Cruz presented around six months into her term, the Special Rapporteur laid out the issues to be addressed and her methodology. The report noted that discrimination related to leprosy still exists at all levels—at the macro level of national policies and laws, at the micro level of community and family, and in between, within institutions and organizations, such as those relating to health services, education and employment. Then the report stressed that an important key to eliminating such structural discrimination is the involvement of those affected by the disease.

Meanwhile, in order to promote the implementation of the P&G, the report noted that while they are not legally binding, the P&G are in line with the human rights standards set out in the Universal Declaration of Human Rights and other human rights instruments, and that the Special Rapporteur would be guided in her work by the relevant conventions, such as those on the rights of persons with disabilities, on the rights of the child, on elimination of discrimination against women and on elimination of racial discrimination.

(ii) The 2019 Thematic Report

In the 2019 thematic report,[29] the Special Rapporteur focuses on "wrongful stereotyping and structural violence against women and children affected by leprosy". She raises the issue of the lack of reliable data on how stereotypes and practices impact the lives of persons affected by leprosy, and how, as a result, they have been historically "dehumanized", particularly through the stigmatizing language of the "leper".

In addition, in order to gain an understanding of the current situation of discrimination, the Special Rapporteur carried out online surveys targeting persons affected by leprosy, their families, health workers and people connected with NGOs. Responses were obtained from 575 people, including those in leprosy high-burden countries such as Brazil, Ethiopia, India, Indonesia, Nepal, Myanmar, Nigeria and the Philippines. These break down into females affected by leprosy (31.9%); males affected by leprosy (33.6%); families of females affected by leprosy (9.8%); families of males affected by leprosy (8%); and health workers/NGO personnel (16.7%).

The survey found that: 1) 42.7% of persons affected by leprosy were isolated from their families and communities; 2) 45.5% said that discrimination was more serious against affected females than affected males; 3) the cause of discrimination against females has a close relationship with poverty (65.9% responded that women are not economically independent); and 4) there are many cases of children being expelled from school, isolated from other pupils, or refused entry.

As reasons why discrimination towards persons affected by leprosy has not disappeared, responses included the following: 1) currently no country has a system for monitoring leprosy and human rights issues; 2) action plans for the appropriate implementation of the P&G have not been set up; and 3) specific measures for amending or abolishing existing discriminatory laws do not exist.

Furthermore, among others, the following recommendations were made: 1) abolish or amend discriminatory laws; 2) involve persons affected by leprosy in decision-making processes that directly affect their lives, and in the process of their implementation; 3) establish reparation measures for persons affected by leprosy, as well as their children, where appropriate; 4) improve monitoring systems for leprosy; 5) empower women affected by leprosy to know their rights; 6) undertake further research into the risk factors that may perpetuate violence against children affected by leprosy; and 7) ensure that children with leprosy-related disabilities participate on an equal basis with others.

(iii) The 2020 Thematic Report

The 2020 thematic report[30] has as its theme the establishment of a "policy framework for rights-based action plans" structured on the following four main axes: 1) adequate standard of living and economic autonomy; 2) non-discrimination, independent living, and inclusion in the community; 3) elimination of stereotypes, and the right to truth and memory; and 4) empowerment.

In considering the policy framework in each of these four areas, the kinds of relationships between the contents of the P&G and various declarations and treaties already adopted or signed by the UN (such as the Universal Declaration of Human Rights, the Convention on the Rights of the Child, the Convention on the Rights of Persons with Disabilities and the Convention on the Elimination of All Forms of Discrimination Against Women), are considered.

Further, by making clear the link between the P&G, which have been adopted by governments but are non-binding, and various binding UN treaties, the Special Rapporteur made the case for there being an obligation to implement the P&G, and introduced several specific examples of success stories in each area.

For example, in regard to "adequate standard of living and economic autonomy", the following examples were given: the establishment of a pension system for persons with disabilities in India and Brazil; livelihood assistance by NGOs for persons affected by leprosy (such as in Mozambique, Niger and Nigeria); and the strengthening of self-care groups in Nepal and elsewhere.

Concerning "non-discrimination, independent living, and inclusion in the community", examples included the Indian government's adoption of a policy of zero discrimination as a result of advocacy on the part of groups of persons affected by leprosy and NGOs in that country.

In regard to "elimination of stereotypes, and the right to truth and memory", examples given included: compensation schemes for former leprosy patients and their families in Japan and Brazil; government operation of a Hansen's disease museum (Japan); government guarantees that residents of former sanatoriums would be allowed to continue to live there (such as in Japan and Taiwan); and NGO support for former patients to return to their home areas (Ghana).

Regarding "empowerment", examples mentioned included: the participation of persons affected by leprosy in the administration of universities in Nepal and Brazil; and support provided by NGOs for women affected by leprosy to fill leadership positions in organizations.

As a final recommendation, in developing and implementing policies that include rights-based action plans to eliminate discrimination against persons affected by leprosy and their families and promote their inclusion in society, the report lists the following measures: 1) respect the rights of persons affected; 2) ensure the participation of persons affected and create a system of governance to guarantee this; 3) collect data on the actual situation of discrimination; 4) build systems to monitor human rights violations; 5) allocate appropriate budgets at the national and state levels; 6) promote international cooperation; and 7) pursue initiatives that work in conjunction with the SDGs.

(iv) The 2021 Thematic Report

The 2021 thematic report[31] described how persons affected by leprosy, who are already excluded from socio-economic systems, are facing unemployment and loss of livelihoods amid the coronavirus pandemic, and are unable to receive the benefits of existing safety nets. The effects extend even to the children of persons affected by leprosy. For instance, many have dropped out of school because they lack access to the necessary technology to move to online learning.

The Special Rapporteur pointed out that it is a serious problem that these conditions have not been accurately understood, and considering that persons affected by leprosy are among the worst affected by the impact of the coronavirus pandemic even among socially disadvantaged groups, the report suggested that governments should consider short-term mitigation action and long-term systemic change.

(v) The 2022 Thematic Report

The focus of the 2022 thematic report[32] is the right to health for persons affected by leprosy and their family members, with the Special Rapporteur noting that the issue is not being addressed in accordance with their actual situation. Current public health policies only emphasize the biomedical aspects of treatment (a disease-centred approach) and do not fully recognize the problem of structural violence—the human rights violations and economic losses that result from contracting a particular disease. In other words, in the case of leprosy, the distribution of multidrug therapy (MDT) to patients free of charge is not the end of the story. For example, services such as reaction management, psychological care, physiotherapy, occupational therapy, group therapy, wound care, surgery, provision of assistive devices and rehabilitation have to be paid for, and persons affected by leprosy also face exclusion from their communities and loss of livelihood. Therefore, when considering the right to health for persons affected by leprosy, a multi-layered interpretation from a broader perspective is required. Although there are civil society organizations working to bridge this gap at the field level, it is difficult for them to reach everyone. The Special Rapporteur concludes that states need to acquire a proper understanding of the right to health for persons affected by leprosy, and must take proactive measures in accordance with their constitutions and international human rights law. Ms. Cruz presented the 2023 Thematic Report in July 2023, which is her final report and examines progress and the remaining challenges in eliminating discrimination against persons affected by leprosy and their family members. However, the report had not yet been published at the time of writing, and is not covered here.

(vi) Official Visits to Brazil and Japan

Ms. Cruz, as Special Rapporteur, made official visits to Brazil and Japan.

(a) Official visit to Brazil

Regarding the official visit to Brazil by the Special Rapporteur in May 2019,[33] her report appreciated the measures taken to eliminate discrimination against persons affected by leprosy and their family members at the institutional level, such as: 1) the fact that discriminatory laws had already been scrapped; 2) the fact that Brazil prohibited discriminatory language, replacing the term "leprosy" (which it recognized as attracting discrimination) with "Hansen's disease" (enacted in 1976, amended in 1995); 3) the fact that laws have been established to compensate persons affected by Hansen's disease who were subjected to compulsory isolation in segregated colonies (2007); and 4) the fact that a law has been adopted for the first time in the world (in Minas Gerais state) granting reparations to the children who were forcibly separated from parents affected by leprosy as part of the compulsory isolation policy (2019).

On the other hand, the report concludes that de facto discrimination endures, for example in the workplace and in educational settings, leading to the conclusion that appropriate implementation of the P&G is needed.

(b) Official visit to Japan

Concerning the official visit to Japan by the Special Rapporteur in February 2020,[34] the report recognized the government's implementation of compensation for persons affected by leprosy and their families through the enactment of new laws following judgments in lawsuits against the government in 2001 and 2019, and the fact that it is conducting awareness-raising activities through the National Hansen's Disease Museum as part of national policy.

At the same time, the report raised some concerns, including: the failure to acknowledge the responsibility of particular professional communities, such as the medical, law, welfare and media communities, for what happened to persons affected by leprosy; the need to reconnect sanatoriums with the surrounding communities; inconsistencies at the local level in the way awareness about Hansen's disease is being raised among schoolchildren; and the need for both the private sector and local governments to give priority to Hansen's disease in their human rights programmes.

Following these visits, the Special Rapporteur made further official visits to Angola (May–June 2022) and Bangladesh (February

2023), but her reports had not yet been published at the time of writing, and are not covered here.

(vii) Extension of the term of the Special Rapporteur

Through a resolution adopted in 2020, Ms. Cruz's term was extended up to October 2023. The resolution requires the Special Rapporteur to present an annual report not only to the Human Rights Council but also to the UNGA.

Ms. Cruz presented a report titled "An unfinished business: discrimination in law against persons affected by leprosy and their family members" at the UNGA Third Committee session in October 2021.[35] In this report, Ms. Cruz said: "The fact that discrimination related to leprosy has become systematised, as well as being a driver for social stigma for the persons affected, encourages others seeing them as non-human, and normalises this." In this report, Ms. Cruz noted that the institutionalization of leprosy-related discrimination has promoted and normalized the stigmatization and dehumanization of persons affected by leprosy. Part of this lies in the existence of discriminatory laws, which the report goes on to analyze.

According to Ms. Cruz, these laws can be broadly divided into eleven areas: 1) laws that violate political rights through prohibition of participation in elections or of holding public office; 2) laws that restrict freedom of movement by prohibiting or restricting the use of public transport; 3) laws that permit divorce on the grounds of leprosy; 4) laws that deny rights to migrants; 5) laws that restrict access to certain jobs; 6) laws that exclude persons from occupying positions of authority in public or private entities, such as universities, or allow for their removal, on grounds of leprosy; 7) laws that enforce compulsory segregation or hospitalization of persons affected by leprosy as part of anti-begging measures; 8) laws that regulate operation of city bodies and public spaces that prohibit persons affected by leprosy from taking up positions or participating in elections; 9) laws relating to prisons that promote compulsory segregation of persons affected by leprosy; 10) laws that maintain segregation as official public health policy for controlling leprosy; and 11) laws, regulations and policies that appear neutral at face value, but that are applied in a manner that discriminates against persons affected by leprosy (indirect discrimination).

At the same time, although it had not been properly verified, the Special Rapporteur expressed the view that the existence of traditional customs and practices that discriminate against persons affected by leprosy cannot be ignored. Moreover, the report proposed that, through establishing comprehensive laws that prohibit discrimination against those affected, including the abolition of discriminatory laws, states should use these as a means of preventing and protecting those affected from discrimination and violence.

At the UN General Assembly in 2022, the Special Rapporteur presented a report titled "Multiple disabilities and fluid self-identification: disability rights of persons affected by leprosy and their family members and how they challenge national legal frameworks",[36] focusing on the rights of persons affected by leprosy and their family members as persons with disabilities. She begins by stating that the issue of leprosy has rarely been addressed at various international conferences on disability rights, and that the realities of the disease have not been adequately verified. On the other hand, while a few states have identified leprosy as a disability issue, she notes that challenges remain. For example: 1) Persons affected are not sufficiently aware of, or do not recognize their rights because they live in remote areas, or are illiterate; 2) Only persons affected by leprosy with visible disabilities are recognized as persons with disabilities, not those with invisible physical impairment such as paralysis or psychosocial impairment stemming from discrimination; and 3) Systemic barriers exist that inhibit the participation of persons affected by leprosy in policymaking and programme development.

The Special Rapporteur believes that persons affected by leprosy should be recognized by states as a group that should enjoy the rights of the Convention on the Rights of Persons with Disabilities (Articles 1 and 2), and that the participation of persons affected by leprosy should be ensured. Her report concludes that states should focus on issues such as: reviewing the eligibility requirements for social protection to ensure access for persons with invisible and

Table 3: Overview of Human Rights Council Resolutions

Resolution 8/13	Resolution 12/7	Resolution 15/10	Resolution 29/5	Resolution 35/9	Resolution 44/6
8th session of Human Rights Council (2–18 June 2008)	12th session of Human Rights Council (14 September–2 October 2009)	15th session of Human Rights Council (13 September–1 October 2010)	29th session of Human Rights Council (15 June–3 July 2015)	35th session of Human Rights Council (6–23 June 2017)	44th session of Human Rights Council (30 June–17 July 2020)
States that leprosy should be recognized as a human rights issue and recommends the following measures: 1) Calls on governments to take measures to eliminate discrimination; 2) Requests OHCHR to include issue of leprosy discrimination in its human rights education and awareness-raising activities; 3) Requests the Human Rights	Requests that the OHCHR collect the views of governments, UN agencies, NGOs and representatives of persons affected by leprosy on the principles and guidelines, and submit a final draft reflecting these views to the 15th session of the Human Rights Council.	Approves the final draft of the principles and guidelines and encourages governments, UN agencies, human rights institutions and stakeholders around the world (schools, hospitals, universities, religious organizations, businesses, the media and NGOs) to give consideration to the principles and guidelines and invites	Mandates the Advisory Committee to review the implementation status of the principles and guidelines and obstacles to such, and submit a report containing suggestions for their wider dissemination and more effective implementation to the 35th session of the Human Rights Council.	Appoints a Special Rapporteur on elimination of discrimination against persons affected by leprosy and their family members for a three-year term, to report annually to the Human Rights Council. States and all relevant stakeholders are to cooperate with the Special Rapporteur in her investigations and the High	Extends the term of the Special Rapporteur for three years, with the Special Rapporteur to continue to report annually to the Human Rights Council and to report also to the UN General Assembly.

Council Advisory Committee to formulate a draft set of principles and guidelines for the elimination of leprosy-related discrimination and submit it by September 2009.

the UN General Assembly to consider the issue of leprosy-related discrimination.

Commissioner and Special Rapporteur are to hold seminars to widely disseminate the principles and guidelines.

Development of the principles and guidelines was overseen by Professor Shigeki Sakamoto of Kobe University (now of Doshisha University), Japan.

A resolution on elimination of discrimination against persons affected by leprosy and their family members, taking note of the principles and guidelines, was adopted unanimously in December the same year.

A record 97 countries co-sponsored the resolution.

The Special Rapporteur is required to start submitting reports from the 38th session of the Human Rights Council in September 2018.

The Special Rapporteur is to report to UN General Assembly from its 76th session in September 2021.

Source: Prepared by the author based on the Resolutions.
At the 53rd session of the Human Rights Council held in July 2023, the term of Special Rapporteur was extended for three years again (A/HRC/RES/53/8).

psychosocial impairments; reviewing the definition of leprosy-related disabilities in line with the human rights model; and recognizing the diversity of persons with disabilities.

5. Mr. Sasakawa's contributions towards the abolition of leprosy discrimination

As has already been discussed, Mr. Sasakawa played a central role in establishing the international consensus that leprosy is a human rights issue. Further, Mr. Sasakawa, over the last almost twenty years, has continued to address leprosy as a human rights issue, and has contributed to achieving some notable milestones, such as the adoption of resolutions at UN Human Rights Council sessions. How was Mr. Sasakawa able to do this? In this section, we will look more closely at the tactics employed by Mr. Sasakawa.

5–1. Effectively grasping "political opportunities"

It is not always easy to reach agreement on issues raised at the Human Rights Council—for example, the human rights situation surrounding the Uygurs—as discussions can be influenced by political conditions in the countries concerned. Leprosy, however, is not a politically charged topic. Not only that, the existence of people still suffering from stigma and discrimination has not been fully recognized, and once the relevant members were made aware of the fact, most were shocked by the seriousness of these issues. Therefore, leprosy is less likely to become a political issue and is more easily accepted by countries as a problem that should be resolved by all humankind.

Indeed, in the process leading to the adoption of the first resolution on elimination of discrimination in 2008, Mr. Sasakawa succeeded in obtaining the support of countries that usually do not welcome initiatives from the government of Japan, such as China and Cuba. In other words, in regard to this matter, there was plenty of room to manoeuvre within the UN political system. Put differently, within the UN, "political opportunities" existed to address leprosy issues.

Mr. Sasakawa's cooperation with the Japanese government is also an important factor. Since only member countries can submit resolutions to the Human Rights Council, it would have been impossible for Mr. Sasakawa as an individual or for the Nippon Foundation to proceed. After Mr. Sasakawa had held his first meeting in 2003 with the then Acting UN High Commissioner for Human Rights Mr. Bertrand Ramcharan, he began building partnerships with the Ministry of Foreign Affairs of the government of Japan and the Permanent Mission of Japan to the International Organizations in Geneva.

The reason why Mr. Sasakawa was able to gain the full cooperation of the government of Japan was influenced by the fact that the Nippon Foundation, the largest private-sector foundation in Japan, already had a track record of collaborating with the government in various fields, and also that as WHO Goodwill Ambassador for Leprosy Elimination, Mr. Sasakawa had travelled all over the world to see the situation for himself and had earned the trust of many of the stakeholders involved with leprosy.

In addition, since Japan had the reputation in the international community of not being as proactive on human rights as Western countries, the government wanted to demonstrate otherwise through its stance on leprosy. Accordingly, while stressing the benefits to both sides of cooperating, Mr. Sasakawa also effectively seized this political opportunity. As evidence of this, in 2007 Mr. Sasakawa was appointed by the government of Japan as its Goodwill Ambassador for the Human Rights of Persons Affected by Leprosy. The fact that Mr. Sasakawa held this title led to the establishment of a smooth cooperative relationship with the government of Japan in the process of a number of resolutions on leprosy discrimination being submitted to and adopted by the Human Rights Council.

5–2. Obtaining support from the beneficiaries—organizations of persons affected by leprosy

As mentioned earlier, many persons affected by leprosy and their family members have long been isolated, neglected or forgotten by society. Moreover, these people differed radically from the usual class of poor people at the bottom of society. That is, while the latter are acknowledged as members of society, albeit on the bottom rung, many persons affected by leprosy were forced to live apart from society and even today still face discrimination in areas such as employment, education and marriage.

In recent years, until the COVID-19 pandemic disrupted leprosy programmes, around 200,000 new cases of leprosy were being reported each year, according to the WHO, and it is estimated that globally there exist tens of millions of people who have recovered from leprosy. Mr. Sasakawa's actions in making the world aware that leprosy is not simply a disease but also a serious human rights problem through his support for the resolutions of the UN Human Rights Council were well received by the beneficiaries, that is, persons affected by leprosy and their family members. Accordingly, Mr. Sasakawa was able to obtain their full support and work closely with organizations around the world that represented them.

5–3. Strategic use of the organizational resources possessed by the Nippon Foundation and the Sasakawa Health Foundation

Mr. Sasakawa made effective use of the organizational resources of the Nippon Foundation, which he chairs, and its sister organization, the Sasakawa Health Foundation, which specializes in leprosy. Since both foundations have a track record of focusing on leprosy for close to half a century, they have built substantial relationships of trust and formed networks with a wide range of actors throughout the world, such as organizations of persons affected by leprosy, NGOs, governments, international bodies, universities and research institutions, and the media.

Foundations generally have a strong tendency to seek tangible results in a short time, and regularly change their policies and areas of support. For example, in the field of public health, there are many diseases that attract more attention than leprosy, such as AIDS, malaria and tuberculosis. Notwithstanding, the two foundations have remained committed to addressing leprosy, while evolving and changing the scope and area of their activities in response to the needs of the times. As a result, they have built up an abundance of "social capital" comprising their relationships of trust and networks with a wide range of actors, and this has been a major contribution to their creating effective cooperative relationships.

Further, both foundations have a solid financial base. As mentioned previously, the Nippon Foundation is the largest private-sector foundation in Japan in terms of its funding, so the fact that sufficient funds can be invested when carrying out a programme of activities is a valuable organizational resource for both foundations.

5–4. Determining clear goals, and framing the central issues

However, even though the two foundations have social capital and a strong financial base, unless those resources are effectively utilized, no progress can be made. Reflecting on this, Mr. Sasakawa proposed framing the leprosy issue as "Leprosy is not only a disease but also a human rights issue"—and strategically collaborated with many different actors, including organizations of persons affected by leprosy (the beneficiaries), experts (such as members of the UN Sub-Commission on the Promotion and Protection of Human Rights and the Human Rights Council Advisory Committee and researchers) and the government of Japan.

Furthermore, he made into central issues the goals to be achieved, such as "adoption of a resolution by the Human Rights Council", "formulation of Principles and Guidelines for the elimination of discrimination", "conducting of research into appropriate implementation of the Principles and Guidelines" and "establishment of a UN Special Rapporteur for the elimination of discrimination against leprosy". He supported investigations through experts, such as Professor Yokota, who for a time served as the Special Rapporteur for the Sub-Commission, and Professor Sakamoto and Mr. Yigezu, who were involved as part of the Human Rights Council Advisory Committee, and through specialized groups such as the IWG, which studied ways to promote the greater spread of the Principles and Guidelines. Based on the results, he sought to justify the need to achieve the goals he had identified as the central issues.

5–5. Summary of tactics and strategies adopted by Mr. Sasakawa in his activities

Below I summarize the tactics utilized by Mr. Sasakawa to bring international public opinion round to the view that leprosy is a human rights issue. First, Mr. Sasakawa proposed that leprosy be framed as a human rights issue and, after gaining the support of organizations of persons affected by leprosy, he also made into central issues the objectives to be obtained, such as "adoption of a resolution by the Human Rights Council" and "the establishment of a UN Special Rapporteur for the elimination of discrimination against leprosy". Then, by strategically mobilizing the resources of the Nippon Foundation and the Sasakawa Health Foundation, he seized political opportunities to effectively approach the UN Human Rights Council and the government of Japan.

The roles played by Mr. Sasakawa in this process can be broadly divided into three:

First, in order to get resolutions adopted by the Human Rights Council, Mr. Sasakawa continuously approached the government of Japan, member countries of the UN Human Rights Council and the members of the Advisory Committee; was consistently involved in the formulation of specific policies and the construction of mechanisms; and exercised an "advocacy and process monitoring function" to seek improvements when problems occurred.

Second, through his support for the survey and research activities of Professor Yokota, Professor Sakamoto, Mr. Yigezu and the IWG, for example, this "information gathering and research function" produced persuasive materials for use in advocacy activities.

Third, and finally, in the process of carrying out the above activities, starting with the five international symposiums on leprosy and human rights, Mr. Sasakawa promoted various mutual alliances by proactively setting up opportunities to join together a wide range of actors, such as organizations of persons affected by leprosy, international NGOs, the government of Japan, universities and research organs. Thus he performed a "catalyst and coordination function" that led to the achievement of the goals that he himself had set.

The fact that Mr. Sasakawa, a private citizen, was able to help bring international public opinion round to the view that leprosy is a human rights issue, leads to the conclusion that the factor behind his success was that he could strategically implement the three functions (advocacy/process monitoring; information gathering/research; catalyst/coordination), based on four clear tactics: effective use of political opportunities; obtaining the support of the beneficiaries; strategic usage of organizational resources; and accurate framing of the central issues.

6. Trends emerging from the activities of Mr. Sasakawa

In this section, I consider the benefits that were brought about by the activities of Mr. Sasakawa that were highlighted in the first section of this chapter.

6–1. Abolition and amendment of discriminatory laws related to leprosy

First, the UNGA resolution and the formulation of the Principles and Guidelines have triggered a growing movement in various countries to investigate discriminatory laws relating to leprosy and to repeal or amend them as a means of promoting the elimination of discrimination related to leprosy.

The International Federation of Anti-Leprosy Associations (ILEP), a federation of fourteen international NGOs working in leprosy, conducted a survey on existing discriminatory laws related to leprosy around the world and found that, as of February 2023, there are 139 such discriminatory laws in twenty-four countries.[37] Of these, 108 are Indian laws, including those at state level.

In light of this, in 2015 the Law Commission of India compiled Report No. 256,[38] identifying the remaining discriminatory laws related to leprosy in India and attaching model draft legislation in the

Eliminating Discrimination against Persons Affected by Leprosy (EDPAL) Bill. It submitted these to the minister of law and justice. The EDPAL Bill is a landmark bill that proposes abolishing all the existing discriminatory laws at one stroke, providing a special pension to persons affected by leprosy in all states, and addressing other matters. Discussion of this bill is not presently advancing in the Indian Parliament. However, between 2016 and 2019, twelve laws in India, including the Lepers Act, were abolished or amended.

In regard to other discriminatory laws related to leprosy, the Marriage Law in China and the Lepers Act in Bangladesh were both abolished in 2011, while in both Sri Lanka and Nepal, the same trend is steadily increasing.[39] For all of these moves, it can be said that the resolutions of the UN, which Mr. Sasakawa played a leading role in bringing about, were the springboard.

6–2. Access to safety nets for affected persons

Second, after the formulation of the Principles and Guidelines, some countries are beginning to provide safety nets for persons affected by leprosy. For example, the twelfth guideline (concerning the right to an adequate standard of living) states that persons affected by leprosy and their family members who are not able to work because of age, illness or disability should be provided with a government pension.

In India, the country with the highest burden of leprosy, the Association of People Affected by Leprosy (APAL), with the strong support of Mr. Sasakawa, took the lead in negotiating with several state governments to create a "special pension system" for persons affected by leprosy with severe disabilities as one means of improving their standard of living. This system is being implemented or considered in at least the Delhi National Capital Region, and in the states of Haryana, Bihar, Uttarakhand, Tamil Nadu, Maharashtra, Uttar Pradesh, Madhya Pradesh, Chhattisgarh and Odisha. The details depend on the state, but in general, recipients are paid around 1,000 to 3,000 rupees per month.[40] In Colombia and Brunei, the same kind of measures are being carried out.[41]

In the state of Minas Gerais in Brazil, a system to compensate children born to persons affected by leprosy who were then forcibly removed from them was set up in 2018. Since the payment provided is insufficient, there is room for improvement; currently, efforts are under way to get the federal government to establish the same kind of compensation system throughout the country.[42]

In the Brazilian state of Maranhão, driven by the partnership that has been formed between MORHAN, the Movement for the Reintegration of Persons Affected by Hansen's Disease, and the Federal Public Defender's Office to monitor discrimination related to leprosy, a National Observatory on Human Rights and Hansen's Disease has been established, as well as a mechanism to constantly monitor discrimination against persons affected by leprosy.

Persons affected by leprosy, even when suffering from severe disabilities, are often excluded from existing safety nets, such as disability or old age pensions, either because governments have not recognized them as disabled, or they are not registered as residents, or their existence itself is not acknowledged.

However, the UN resolutions and the establishment of the P&G have led to change. For example, in India, with the enactment of the 2016 Rights of Persons with Disabilities Act, leprosy was recognized as a disability for the first time. As a result, disability cards began to be distributed to persons affected by leprosy, and it became possible for them to receive the same benefits as other disabled persons.

From a global perspective, it is still rare for persons affected by leprosy to be guaranteed the same rights as other persons with disabilities; hence, the above-mentioned development can be described as epoch-making. Currently, organizations of persons affected by leprosy and NGOs in various parts of the world are endeavouring to see this development spread to other countries.

6–3. A shift in the policies of the WHO and national governments

The WHO, which has played a central role in combatting leprosy as a disease, has also begun to address the problem of discrimination and stigma. In 2011, after holding consultations with stakeholders including persons affected by leprosy, the WHO published

Guidelines for strengthening participation of persons affected by leprosy in leprosy services.[43] Moreover, the Global Leprosy Programme (GLP), which oversees leprosy control at the WHO, has issued a global leprosy strategy document every five years since 2006. In *Global Leprosy Strategy 2016–2020: Accelerating towards a leprosy-free world*,[44] one of the four elements of its vision was "Zero leprosy and discrimination", and it recommended that countries tackle both medical and social aspects of the disease. This policy is also being followed in *Towards Zero Leprosy: Global Leprosy (Hansen's disease) Strategy 2021–2030*, released in 2021.[45]

Since each country usually determines its leprosy policy based on the GLP strategy, addressing issues of stigma and discrimination in parallel with tackling the disease has become mainstream in national leprosy programmes. Meanwhile, among international NGOs affiliated with ILEP, mentioned earlier, the practice of addressing leprosy from both medical and social perspectives has taken root at the grassroots level, as seen in the requirement to include discrimination in the curriculum when training medical personnel in case detection.

6–4. Empowerment of persons affected by leprosy

The adoption of UN resolutions and formulation of the Principles and Guidelines can also be seen as an important benefit that contributed to the empowerment of persons affected by leprosy. As a result of the international community's recognition of the need to eliminate discrimination against persons affected by leprosy and their family members, many persons affected by leprosy have raised their voices, and there has been a growing movement to establish organizations of persons affected by leprosy in many parts of the world.

According to a survey carried out by Ms. Paula Brandao, who serves as a volunteer for MORHAN, a movement for the reintegration of persons affected by Hansen's disease in Brazil, forty-nine organizations of persons affected by leprosy have been established in twenty-seven countries (counting only those that have been verified). Besides these, there are also many self-help groups throughout the world made up of persons affected by leprosy that are not formally organized.

At the Global Forum of People's Organizations on Hansen's Disease organized by the Nippon Foundation and the Sasakawa Health Foundation in Manila, the Philippines, in September 2019, with Mr. Sasakawa at its centre, eighty persons affected by leprosy from eighteen countries gathered to discuss promoting participation of persons affected by leprosy in leprosy services and their empowerment. In the Manila Declaration[46] adopted at the end of the conference, delegates agreed that networks of persons affected by leprosy should be strengthened at the global level. In November 2022, a 2nd Global Forum took place in Hyderabad, India, with around 100 representatives of people's organizations from twenty-one countries participating. Meanwhile, for those tackling Neglected Tropical Diseases (NTDs), which comprise twenty diseases including leprosy, the elimination of discrimination against persons affected by these diseases has become an important theme, with persons affected by leprosy taking the lead.

In this way, the adoption of the UN resolutions and the formulation of the Principles and Guidelines, with Mr. Sasakawa playing a central role, has led to increased activity on abolishing discriminatory laws in many countries, greater access to safety nets for persons affected by leprosy, realization of a policy shift to include measures to resolve discrimination and stigma in the leprosy strategies of the WHO and national governments, and the promotion of the empowerment of persons affected by leprosy all over the world.

7. Lessons to be learned beyond leprosy issues

As described above, it is a fact that Mr. Sasakawa's wide-ranging activities have made a major contribution to spreading a common awareness that discrimination against persons affected by leprosy and their family members is a human rights issue, and that the international community and governments should work for its elimination. At the same time, another achievement of Mr. Sasakawa's, as explained below, is that he has provided many suggestions which can help us address future issues on a more global level, beyond the framework of the elimination of discrimination against leprosy.

7–1. Embodying the role of the non-profit sector as a major actor in global governance

The first implication embodies the role that the non-profit sector can play as a major actor in global governance. The fact that through the adoption of as many as six resolutions by the UN Human Rights Council an international awareness that leprosy is a human rights issue has been established, and a mechanism developed for the international community to work sustainably to resolve this issue, would have been unthinkable without the achievements of Mr. Sasakawa.

As background to this, several factors contributed greatly to these results. Through the Nippon Foundation and the Sasakawa Health Foundation, Mr. Sasakawa grasped political opportunities; obtained the support of beneficiaries; mobilized the organizational resources possessed by the two foundations; came up with the tactic of making a central issue of the necessity for the international community to address leprosy; and effectively implemented the functions of advocacy/process monitoring, information gathering/research and catalyst/coordination.

It is no exaggeration to say that the contributions made by Mr. Sasakawa, a representative of a private non-profit organization, are comparable to other examples in which the non-profit sector has played an important role in the international community, such as in achieving the Anti-Personnel Mine Ban Convention and the Convention on Cluster Munitions. He has provided an important model for considering the roles the non-profit sector can play in solving other social issues in the future.

7–2. Demonstrating measures towards the "realization of a society where no one is left behind"

The second implication involves the fact that Mr. Sasakawa has consistently, from start to finish, embodied the core principle of the SDGs, namely, "the realization of a society where no one is left behind". As mentioned earlier, Mr. Sasakawa has likened the fight against leprosy to the two wheels of a motorcycle, with the front wheel symbolizing treating the disease, and the back wheel representing activities to eliminate discrimination, and stressed that both wheels need to be turning at the same speed. This will be of great help in the fight against other infectious diseases, particularly when it comes to achieving Goal 3 (Good Health and Well-Being) of the SDGs and especially 3–3, to end AIDS, tuberculosis, malaria and NTDs, and combat hepatitis, water-borne diseases and other communicable diseases by 2030.

In particular, when considering measures against infectious diseases, this means not simply curing the disease, but also giving due consideration to the human rights of affected persons. This can clearly be seen, for example, in relation to the recent coronavirus pandemic. Accordingly, Mr. Sasakawa's example in addressing leprosy as a human rights issue can provide an effective model for the international community when considering other infectious disease measures. Moreover, many persons affected by leprosy are the most vulnerable of all socially disadvantaged people, with their very existence having been long forgotten.

Mr. Sasakawa enabled their human rights to be acknowledged by the international community, provided them with opportunities to make themselves heard in the international community, and contributed to constructing a mechanism to sustainably address leprosy as a human rights issue. This can be seen as a pioneering example, demonstrating what it means to aim for a society in which "no one is left behind", as advocated in the SDGs, and how to realize it.

In conclusion

As outlined above, Mr. Sasakawa has already achieved a great deal (see Table 4). However, he is definitely not satisfied with the current state of affairs. As evidence for this, I would like to end here by quoting from Mr. Sasakawa's remarks in his message for the 100th issue of the *WHO Goodwill Ambassador's Newsletter for the Elimination of Leprosy* (now the *WHO Goodwill Ambassador's Leprosy Bulletin*), which has been published since 2003:

My dream is for an inclusive society—one in which not only persons affected by leprosy but all vulnerable groups have a place. Hence my journey continues. Zero leprosy and zero discrimination may not be achieved in my lifetime, but I will do my best to help us get there.[47]

The true strength of Mr. Sasakawa is his passion, which still overflows even though he is now over eighty years old, his commitment to on-site activities and his attitude of never giving up trying to achieve his goals. This is what we must all learn equally if we are to solve social issues in the future.

Table 4: The main activities of Mr. Sasakawa in addressing leprosy and human rights issues [*NOTE: Not all activities listed here are Mr. Sasakawa's activities; his activities are shown in roman type, all others in italics*]

2001	
January	Appointed as GAEL Special Ambassador
October	Gives keynote speech on leprosy and human rights at the 5th Forum 2000 Conference
2003	
July	Has meeting with Mr. Bertrand Ramcharan, Acting UN High Commissioner for Human Rights; they discuss leprosy and human rights issues
August	Holds a side event at the 55th session of the UN Sub-Commission on the Protection and Promotion of Human Rights Meets with UN Special Rapporteur on "Right to Health" Paul Hunt, a professor at University of Essex
2004	
March	As well as organizing a side event at the 60th plenary session of the UN Commission on Human Rights, announces the first oral statement on leprosy and human rights

May	Organizes explanatory meeting for the UN High Commissioner for Human Rights staff Appointed as the WHO Leprosy Elimination Ambassador
July	*During the holding of the 56th session of the UN Sub-Commission on the Protection and Promotion of Human Rights, hosts luncheon discussion meeting for Sub-Commission members (attended by 22 of 26). The Sub-Commission appoints Mr. Yozo Yokota as Special Rapporteur to conduct surveys on "the issue of discrimination against leprosy sufferers and their families" and adopts a resolution for him to present a preliminary report at their next yearly meeting*
September	Writes an article stating the need to tackle leprosy as a human rights issue, which is featured in the *International Herald Tribune*
November	Meets in Tokyo the newly appointed UN High Commissioner for Human Rights, Ms. Louise Arbour
2005	
August	*At the 57th session of the UN Sub-Commission on the Protection and Promotion of Human Rights, Special Rapporteur Yokota presents the survey results, and the Sub-Commission adopts a resolution promoting the elimination of leprosy discrimination* Gives the floor to persons affected by leprosy from India, Nepal and Ghana during oral statements (the first time that persons affected have addressed a session of the Sub-Commission)
2006	
January	Holds the first annual Global Appeal for the elimination of stigma and discrimination against persons affected by leprosy (the appeal is launched each year on or near World Leprosy Day at the end of January)

March	*The UN Human Rights Council is established following the dissolution of the UN Commission on Human Rights*
August	*At the 58th session of the UN Sub-Commission on the Promotion and Protection of Human Rights, Professor Yokota again submits a report, and the Sub-Commission adopts a resolution supporting its contents (subsequently, the Sub-Commission is disbanded)*
September	In conjunction with the 2nd session of the Human Rights Council, sends a letter to each member urging them to respect the resolutions on leprosy adopted by the Sub-Commission *The government of Japan issues a statement seeking follow-up on the resolutions on leprosy adopted by the Sub-Commission*
2007	
September	Is appointed Goodwill Ambassador for the Human Rights of Persons Affected by Leprosy, by the government of Japan Submits a written request on leprosy and human rights to all members of the Human Rights Council and organizes a side event and reception
2008	
May	Visits the Permanent Missions of 27 countries to the International Organizations in Geneva, requesting their understanding and cooperation in regard to the resolutions on leprosy
June	*At the 8th session of the UN Human Rights Council, a resolution on elimination of discrimination against persons affected by leprosy and their family members is adopted by the Council for the first time (A/HRC/RES/8/13)*
August	*At the 1st session of the Human Rights Advisory Committee, Shigeki Sakamoto, professor at Kobe University, is nominated to produce a report on the compilation of the draft*

	"Principles and Guidelines for the elimination of discrimination against persons affected by leprosy and their family members"
2009	
January	*An official consultation on leprosy and human rights—the first such meeting ever held at the European headquarters of the UN—takes place in Geneva*
October	*At the 12th session of the UN Human Rights Council, Professor Sakamoto submits the draft P&G, and a second resolution on leprosy is adopted (A/HRC/RES/12/7)*
2010	
October	*At the 15th session of the UN Human Rights Council, a third resolution on leprosy is adopted, accompanied by the P&G (A/HRC/RES/15/10)*
December	*The above resolution is unanimously adopted at the 65th UN General Assembly*
2012	
January	*Holding of 1st Leprosy and Human Rights Symposium (Rio de Janeiro, Brazil)*
	Establishment of International Working Group on Leprosy and Human Rights (IWG)
October	*Holding of 2nd Leprosy and Human Rights Symposium (New Delhi, India)*
2013	
September	*Holding of 3rd Leprosy and Human Rights Symposium (Addis Ababa, Ethiopia)*
2014	
November	*Holding of 4th Leprosy and Human Rights Symposium (Rabat, Morocco)*

2015	
June July	*Holding of 5th Leprosy and Human Rights Symposium (Geneva, Switzerland)* *IWG report submitted to the Human Rights Council Advisory Committee* *The 29th session of the UN Human Rights Council adopts a fourth resolution on leprosy (A/HRC/RES/29/5)*
August	*The 15th session of the UN Human Rights Council Advisory Committee names Mr. Imeru Tamrat Yigezu of Ethiopia to compile a report surveying the state of implementation of the P&G*
2017	
July	*Mr. Yigezu submits report to the 35th session of the UN Human Rights Council* *The UN Human Rights Council adopts a fifth resolution on leprosy and establishes the position of Special Rapporteur on leprosy (A/HRC/RES/35/9)*
September	*The 36th session of the UN Human Rights Council names Ms. Alice Cruz as the Special Rapporteur for the Elimination of Leprosy Discrimination*
2018	
June	*Special Rapporteur submits first report at the 38th session of the UN Human Rights Council*
2019	
May	*Official visit to Brazil by Special Rapporteur*
June	*Special Rapporteur submits second report at the 41st session of the UN Human Rights Council*
September	*The Nippon Foundation and the Sasakawa Health Foundation hold Global Forum of People's Organizations on Hansen's Disease (Manila, the Philippines)*

2020	
February	*Official visit to Japan by Special Rapporteur, meets with Mr. Sasakawa*
July	*Special Rapporteur submits third report at the 44th session of the UN Human Rights Council* *The 44th session of the Human Rights Council adopts a sixth resolution on leprosy; the term of the Special Rapporteur is extended for a further three years (A/HR/RES/44/6)*
2021	
June	*Special Rapporteur submits 4th report at the 47th session of the UN Human Rights Council*
October	*Special Rapporteur presents 1st report at the 76th session of the UN General Assembly*
2022	
April	*Official visit to Angola by Special Rapporteur*
June	*Special Rapporteur submits 5th report at the 50th session of the UN Human Rights Council*
October	*Special Rapporteur presents 1st report at the 77th session of UN General Assembly*
November	*The Nippon Foundation and Sasakawa Health Foundation hold 2nd Global Forum of People's Organizations on Hansen's Disease (Hyderabad, India)*
2023	
February	*Official visit to Bangladesh by Special Rapporteur*
July	*At the 53rd session of Human Rights Council, the term of Special Rapporteur is extended for three years again (A/HRC/RES/53/8)*

4

TOWARDS THE ESTABLISHMENT OF THE
RIGHTS OF THE PRIMARY STAKEHOLDERS

Artur Custódio

It is an honour to write about the WHO Goodwill Ambassador for Leprosy Elimination, Mr. Yohei Sasakawa, and it is even more challenging to write about the impact of his influence in advocating for people affected by Hansen's disease globally. In some situations, "measuring impact" becomes a very difficult task. This is one of them: how to talk about this human being and his career that cannot be expressed in mathematical calculations, tables, graphs, scales or formulas.

Before starting this chapter, which I prefer to write in the first person, it is necessary to point out where I am coming from. In 1980, when I was a teenager, I began to carry out volunteer work in Hansen's disease for religious reasons. At the end of 1985, after getting a job in the public sector with the Health Department of the State of Rio de Janeiro, I encountered the Movement for the Reintegration of Persons Affected by Hansen's Disease (MORHAN) in Petrópolis. Founded in 1981, MORHAN was one of the first movements of people affected by Hansen's disease in the world, along with similar organizations in Japan and Korea. Their way of acting and the philosophy of this movement enchanted me and encouraged me to join as a volunteer.

From this experience, and from the perspective of someone who has essentially lived and breathed this cause for so many decades, I shall proceed to give my assessment of the progress that the actions developed by Mr. Sasakawa and his organization have helped to bring about, whether within MORHAN, in Brazil or around the world. Later, I shall draw parallels between different countries and cultures.

With no aspiration to be historically or academically accurate, and with a strong emotional charge, this brief account does not exhaust the scope of Mr. Sasakawa's actions in the world. An entire book would not do justice to the impact of each of his actions in Brazil, or to the transformative effects that his actions have had in the territories and in the lives of each person affected by the disease and their family members—and it is necessary to emphasize that we understand how important it has been to involve the family at all times in these actions, and include them in the care required.

In 1990, when we were still celebrating the overthrow of the last discriminatory law related to Hansen's disease in Brazil and were working hard to give MORHAN leverage with the government of the day, one of our leaders and founders, Mr. Francisco Augusto "Bacurau", assigned me the mission of preparing for his trip to the 14th International Leprosy Congress in Orlando, Florida, in 1993. On his return, he reported on his participation in the Congress and his meeting with other leaders of persons affected by Hansen's disease from different countries, with whom he had discussed a proposal for the internationalization of the movement. Among other ideas, he suggested that pictures of persons affected by the disease should no longer be used in public campaigns as they contributed to the stigmatization of the disease.

It was in this conversation with him that I first heard Mr. Sasakawa's name. The reports indicated that he was a person whose actions were less oriented towards providing care and more focused on helping people to be the protagonists in the process of transforming their lives.

In 1994, following the expressed wish of people affected by Hansen's disease, we held a meeting in Petrópolis to found IDEA—the International Association for Integration, Dignity and Economic Advancement. This meeting indirectly marked the first support given to MORHAN by the Nippon Foundation (TNF), the organization led by Mr. Sasakawa. The status of IDEA worldwide was based on the statutes of MORHAN, which at that time was in its thirteenth year. From that year onwards, I would hear Mr. Sasakawa's name almost daily and would have the privilege of being able to closely follow some of his achievements.

Now, a brief return to our timeline. In the late 1980s and early 1990s, I was working as a health worker in Nova Iguaçu, a city in the state of Rio de Janeiro, with many of its inhabitants coming from the north and northeast of Brazil in search of better opportunities. It was a time when Hansen's disease was highly endemic in that municipality. During this period, I was able to follow the trajectory and experiences of patients diagnosed with Hansen's disease who were still being treated with monotherapy over many years. One of my duties was to go to the homes of those who had given up on treatment and try to convince them to resume, as well as helping in the discovery of new cases among family members. It was at that time that multidrug therapy (MDT) was introduced as the treatment for the disease—not new drugs, but a combination of three existing drugs. In the early days, we had to manually package the medicines, which arrived separately, in plastic bags. We had to pack one of the drugs in flour so that the pills wouldn't melt and stick together. Problems with the quality of the medication—and sometimes even the lack of medication altogether—were common.

This was the reality of the health services in relation to Hansen's disease until 1995, when blister packs of MDT donated by the Nippon Foundation were introduced to Brazil. Working with MORHAN, I could see the impact of this donation at the national level through my interactions with government and also at the front lines of caring for people with the disease. I witnessed the transformation that this brought to the life of each person who started their treatment. This new way of distributing MDT was less time-consuming, involved fewer people, cut down on wastage, and made it possible to quickly and regularly reach people undergoing treatment. As a result, the supply and quality of the medicine improved and it was easier to control stocks and monitor treatment and defaulters. It also meant greater dignity and care for the patient.

From that year, IDEA, supported by Mr. Sasakawa's foundation, began a worldwide expansion, holding meetings to raise awareness, exchange experiences and to provide training. It was in Spain, at one of these meetings, held in the former colony of Fontilles, that I was able to have closer contact with TNF, despite the language barrier. We had our first direct dialogue, facilitated by Ms. Kay Yamaguchi of the Sasakawa Memorial Health Foundation (now known as the Sasakawa Health Foundation). At this meeting, the reports from people affected by Hansen's disease were impressive, and reflected a mixture of gratitude and admiration for Mr. Sasakawa's achievements around the world.

There, in the midst of the development of IDEA, and with the assistance of the Sasakawa Health Foundation, a form of support that had never existed before for organizations in the field of Hansen's disease was born. As it developed, it would give space to and amplify the voices of people affected by Hansen's disease.

Hansen's disease has a very strong social impact that is related to social and economic differences and a lack of human rights. Also, because it is associated with the structural stigma existing in almost all cultures, it generates and perpetuates a cycle of poverty, misery and social invisibility. What Mr. Sasakawa, in a visionary way, was already doing at that time, was to provide instruments of empowerment for people with the disease, so that instead of doctors speaking on their behalf, they could exercise their own power of speech and be the protagonists in their struggles to bring about necessary changes to the way the disease was being tackled in their countries and to the policies of the WHO itself.

There were several international events organized by IDEA with the support of the Nippon Foundation in which MORHAN directors participated. Mr. Bacurau, Mr. Antônio Borges, Ms. Valdenora Rodrigues, Mr. Thiago Flores, Mr. Edimilson Picanço, Mr. Faustino Pinto, Ms. Zilda Borges, Ms. Francisca Barros, and many other leaders among persons affected in Brazil, felt able to conquer the world and make their voices and demands heard.

The International Leprosy Congress, previously attended only by doctors and scientists, started to see other knowledge introduced. Professionals and governments had to listen to the experiences of those who felt, on their own skin, in the sequelae and in their lives, the expression of social stigma and the burden of living with this disease every day. The corridors of the UN, WHO, UNESCO and other international organizations began to receive groups of people who came from the most marginalized and feared sections of society in world history.

Over a five-year period from 1995 to 1999, TNF donated MDT all over the world, millions of people were cured and, as a consequence, many thousands of people did not develop Hansen's disease sequelae. Further, the speed of transmission of the disease was reduced as a result of early access to medicine, the intensification of training and the dissemination of information about the disease. The drug donations were taken over by Novartis and Novartis Foundation from the year 2000. Fortunately, this was not the end of Mr. Sasakawa's involvement, as he knew there were still many more challenges to be overcome to eliminate the disease.

In 2001, Mr. Sasakawa was appointed Goodwill Ambassador for Leprosy Elimination—recognition by the World Health Organization of his outstanding work in global public health. As Goodwill Ambassador he began a new round of travel—a great world marathon—visiting dozens of countries to meet with leaders on his mission to strengthen the fight against Hansen's disease and defend people affected by the disease.

Thousands of people affected by Hansen's disease, leading health professionals, governmental and non-governmental leaders, artists and other partners, including the media, heard his message. In fact, it is important to talk especially about the media, a sector for whom Hansen's disease was an invisible, forgotten disease. On his travels as WHO Goodwill Ambassador, Mr. Sasakawa was always careful to generate interest in the topic, based on his visits and messages. And, more than that, the way he related to the media was always faithful to the principle of portraying people affected by the disease as protagonists, seeking to spotlight them as the citizens they are, and not as objects of charity.

A particularly striking episode during this phase took place in 2004 when, already preparing a new strategy that would be launched in January 2006 to seek support from society and government, Mr. Sasakawa arrived in Brazil. In partnership with MORHAN, he met with the then president of the republic Luiz Inácio Lula da Silva and invited him to be part of a global appeal against the stigma related to Hansen's disease. The invitation was promptly accepted by Brazil's leader.

Despite having had several brief encounters with Mr. Sasakawa at events held in other countries, it was during this visit to Brazil in 2004 that, for the first time, I was able to have a longer conversation with him. His commitment to the cause and care for people, his restless mind and his eagerness to change the world impressed me deeply. I've never forgotten his expression, his firm voice and his certainty that he was on the right path—standing by society's most forgotten people, making sure they would no longer be overlooked, no longer left behind.

It was a conversation that not only allowed me to learn a little more about the man I already admired, but also to hear his story in his own words. The people around us were in a hurry because there was a schedule to keep, but I wanted to learn more and more, and he shared his knowledge with me thoughtfully and generously.

I heard from him the story of how he became involved in the fight against Hansen's disease. In 1965, as a young man, he accompanied his father, Mr. Ryoichi Sasakawa, the founder of TNF, on a trip to South Korea, during which they visited a Hansen's disease hospital. Seeing the way his father moved among the patients, offering words of encouragement, decided him on the path he wanted his own life to take. Hansen's disease would then become his life's work—years dedicated to positioning persons affected by the disease at the centre of policy decisions regarding them, in order to restore their dignity.

The effects and ramifications of that conversation were immediate. His harmony with the basic needs of people with the disease and his enterprising and humanitarian outlook marked the beginning of a partnership of brothers that would last until today. From that moment on, MORHAN's dialogue with the Nippon Foundation became direct, without intermediaries.

Still in 2004, in the wake of Mr. Sasakawa's visit to Brazil and with the active involvement of the Brazilian government in the cause, we had the first national meeting of residents of former Hansen's disease colonies, which resulted in 127 proposals taken to President Lula da Silva. In early 2005, we counted on the Goodwill Ambassador's support and presence at an international seminar in Rio de Janeiro on Hansen's disease and human rights, in which members of the UN Sub-Commission on the Promotion and Protection of Human Rights participated. This introduced us to another initiative of the Nippon Foundation: the framing of the disease as an issue of human rights. Mr. Sasakawa showed another of his characteristics: the ability to build bridges. We were introduced to Professor Yozo Yokota, who, together with TNF, was paving the way for a human rights approach that would prove to be a milestone in strategies for coping with the disease.

Also in 2005, we had Mr. Sasakawa's support, through TNF, for one of our most important projects, TELEHANSEN: a free telephone hotline for the entire population providing information on any question about Hansen's disease. Over the years, this has served as a model project for listening to people affected by Hansen's disease that has guided many other MORHAN strategies.

In 2006, another international strategy was put into practice, with the potential to impact on strengthening national and patient-based organizations around the world. This was the first Global Appeal, issued from New Delhi, India, endorsed by a group of world leaders (including Brazil's President Lula da Silva) and Nobel Peace Prize winners, and led by Mr. Sasakawa. Thereafter, on or near every World Hansen's Disease Day on the last Sunday of January, a new Global Appeal is launched, calling for an end to stigma and discrimination against persons affected by Hansen's disease. We are confident that the appeal will continue to be issued

111

until it is no longer necessary, when we are at the dawn of a world free from Hansen's disease and, above all, free from prejudice. Each Global Appeal, although signed by different individuals and organizations, has had the same objective: the restoration of dignity and human rights of people affected by Hansen's disease. In Brazil, the impact of each appeal has varied according to which organization has endorsed it.

The importance of shining a spotlight on persons affected by Hansen's disease at the national level makes the Global Appeal reverberate in every country, strengthening the fight against the disease and discrimination and impacting local politics. This has undoubtedly been a fundamental strategy to combat stigma and address the violations of people's human rights, in addition to supporting the discussions between governments, civil society organizations and transnational bodies. The range and scope of those partnering with the Global Appeal is impressive, representing fields such as health, religion, education, human rights, employment and para sport, and highlighting areas where people affected by Hansen's disease face daily difficulties due to prejudice and discrimination.

Returning to the specific discussion of human rights, in 2003 the Ambassador approached the Office of the UN High Commissioner for Human Rights, and from this initial encounter, through his foundation, began to lay the groundwork for a UN resolution on ending Hansen's disease-related discrimination. Over the next several years, a number of meetings were held with the participation of human rights experts and leaders of movements of people affected by Hansen's disease, among others. In December 2010, Mr. Sasakawa's efforts were crowned with success when the UN General Assembly adopted a resolution on elimination of discrimination against persons affected by leprosy and their family members, accompanied by principles and guidelines (P&G).

But for the Goodwill Ambassador this was not enough; it was necessary to encourage member states to follow through on the resolution and implement the principles and guidelines. From 2012, several regional international symposiums were held in order to help raise awareness of the principles and guidelines, especially among social movements of people affected, and encourage governments to comply with them.

Subsequently, in 2017, acting in the interests of persons affected by Hansen's disease, Mr. Sasakawa lobbied successfully for the UN Human Rights Council to appoint a Special Rapporteur on the Elimination of Discrimination against Persons Affected by Leprosy and their Family Members. Dr. Alice Cruz, the Special Rapporteur, is now in her second term, building a human rights approach to Hansen's disease and promoting the effective recognition of people affected by the disease as subjects of rights, linking this recognition to their exercise of the right to participate in society.

Mr. Sasakawa has worked tirelessly for the global elimination of Hansen's disease, supported meetings and events through his foundation, and insisted on the need for persons affected by Hansen's disease to be active participants—"Nothing about us, without us", in the mantra of the disability movement. Little by little, with a lot of advocacy and diplomacy, he has been able to break down barriers and strengthen their presence.

Breaking down barriers has not been easy, as persons affected by Hansen's disease tend to come from the most vulnerable economic strata of society, making it harder for them to be heard and even to speak out. The effects of stigma, prejudice and discrimination are constantly underestimated in public policies, even within the WHO.

Recent studies from the University of Birmingham in England point to delays of more than ten years in the diagnosis of Hansen's disease cases in Brazil. According to the researchers from the university, there are strong indications that the reduction of the social stigma associated with this disease could encourage people affected by Hansen's disease in Brazil to seek early treatment for their condition. The study, which focused on three reference clinics in different Brazilian states, found that people who suspected they had symptoms of the disease but feared being discriminated against by their communities were ten times more likely to delay seeking care for their symptoms.

Mr. Sasakawa was and continues to be a strong advocate for the participation of persons affected by Hansen's disease in defining the strategies, norms and policies to be adopted. In 2011, the WHO issued guidelines on strengthening the participation of persons affected by leprosy in leprosy services, signalling that the WHO was starting, even if still in an incipient way, to consult persons affected and their organizations. In 2016, the WHO made the "third pillar" of its *Global Leprosy Strategy 2016–2020* eliminating discrimination and promoting the inclusion of people affected by Hansen's disease.

In 2015, with the support of TNF, people affected by Hansen's disease from MORHAN talked to Pope Francis at the Vatican, asking that the word "leprosy" and the word "leper" no longer be used to refer to the disease and the people afflicted. Also at this meeting, the then Executive Director of TNF, Mr. Tatsuya Tanami, delivered a letter from Mr. Sasakawa that culminated a year later, in June 2016, with the holding of an international symposium at the Vatican with TNF and other partners, religious leaders from different faiths, and organizations of persons affected by Hansen's disease. The event was part of the actions taking place during the year designated by the Catholic Church as the Extraordinary Jubilee of Mercy. At a public Mass before the symposium, Mr. Sasakawa personally delivered a letter to the Pope and directly conveyed to him his views on the injustice caused by discrimination related to Hansen's disease.

Now, every year, the Pope transmits messages to more than 1.2 billion members of the Catholic Church, in which he salutes the sick, family members, workers, and communities, and urges all Catholics to act in the fight against prejudice.

Mr. Sasakawa has concentrated his efforts on those countries with the highest incidence of Hansen's disease, on those that still have laws and strong discriminatory attitudes, and also on those that have reached the elimination threshold at the national level, but that have pockets of high endemicity that are overlooked by governments. This has made Brazil and India almost permanent fixtures on Mr. Sasakawa's agenda. Despite my best efforts, I cannot begin to count how many times Mr. Sasakawa has been present at activities organized by MORHAN. There have been numerous interactions with artists and the press, and involvement in other

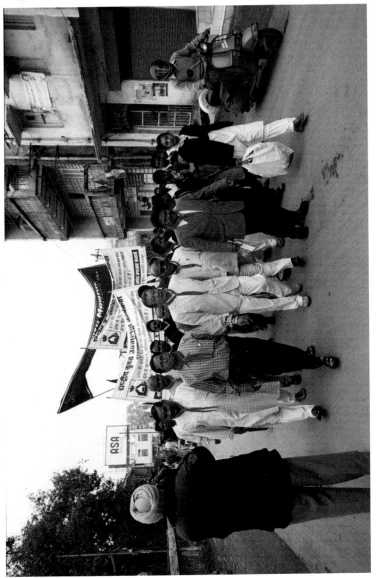

1. Mr. Sasakawa marching with the Minister of Health for the leprosy elimination campaign in Chhattisgarh, India, January 2004.

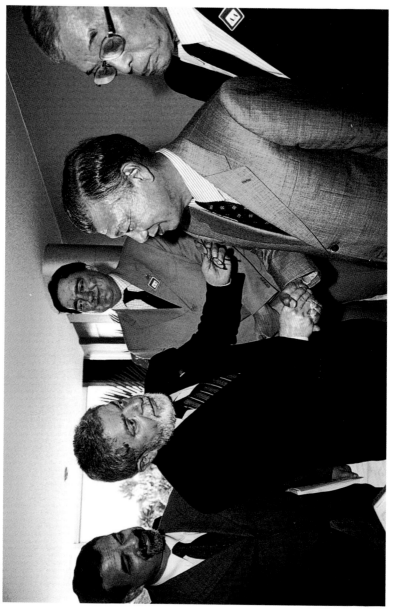

2. Meeting with President Lula da Silva in Brazil, July 2004.

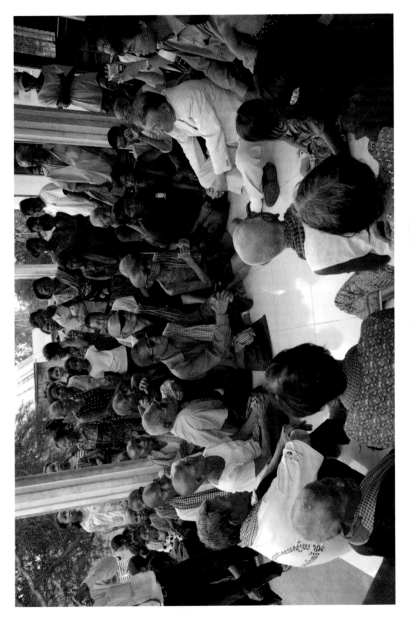

3. Meeting with people in Treng village, Cambodia, February 2008.

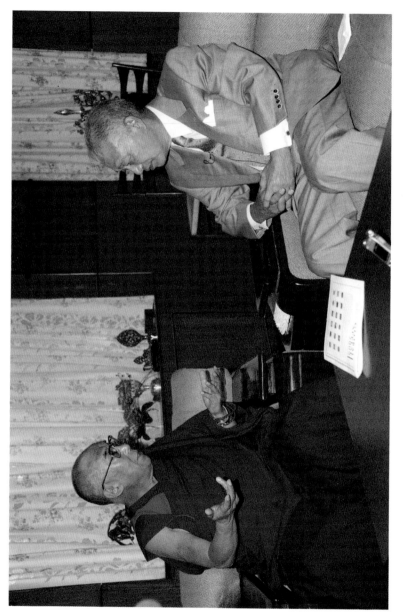

4. Meeting with the Dalai Lama in Himachal Pradesh, India, August 2012.

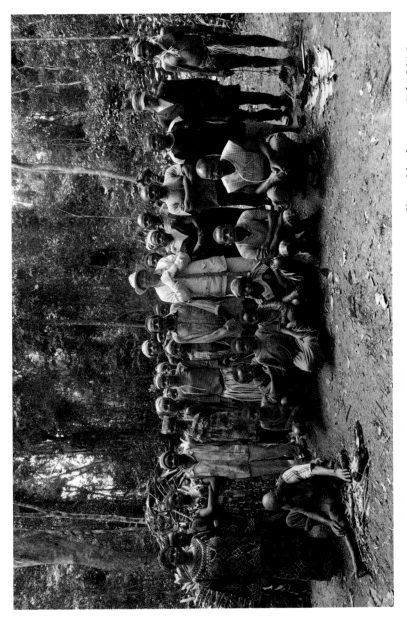

5. Visiting a tribe living in the forest of Cameroon to meet persons affected by leprosy, July 2016.

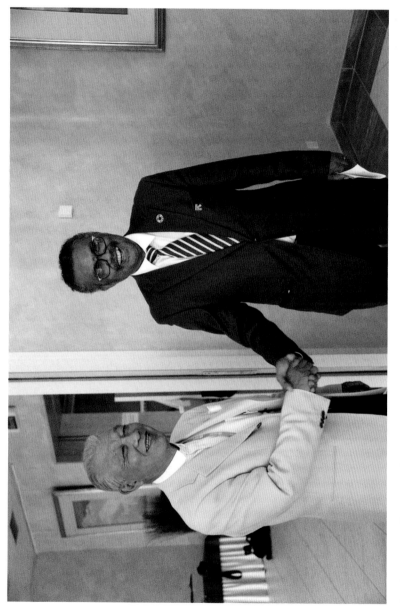

6. Meeting with Dr. Tedros, Director-General of the WHO, at WHO headquarters, May 2018.

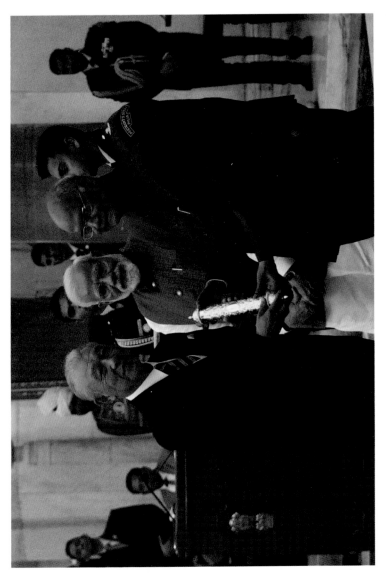

7. At the International Gandhi Peace Prize ceremony with Prime Minister Modi (centre) and former President Kovind (right), February 2019.

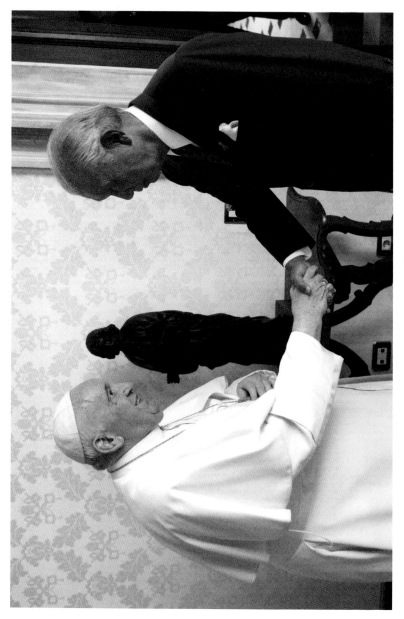

8. Meeting with Pope Francis at the Vatican, January 2023. © Vatican Media.

activities, in which he firmly defended the inclusion of MORHAN in decision-making spaces, even if he sometimes put himself in difficult situations from a diplomatic standpoint. What prevailed in his conduct was his fidelity to the principle of defending people affected and strengthening their organizations. He also joined MORHAN's struggles, such as the fight to have the separation of children from their parents because of Hansen's disease recognized as a crime by the state.

I remember that on at least three occasions Mr. Sasakawa gave me advice and strongly encouraged me not to give up the fight. This is a personal aspect of this world leader that is not likely to appear in scientific or historical research, but which needs to be reported—the care that defines his actions from macro world politics to the field of the individual. On one of these occasions, I was exhausted from the struggle and on the verge of giving up on volunteer militancy, but after a conversation with him I left re-energized to continue.

The progress of Hansen's disease elimination in some countries has brought new issues to be explored and resolved. In this way, allying associations of people affected by Hansen's disease with associations of people with disabilities, respecting some specificities, can be an important strategy to guarantee rehabilitation and economic and social security rights, which has been another strategy adopted by Mr. Sasakawa.

As you can see, the Ambassador's actions advance in several fields simultaneously. When he realizes there is a problem to solve, he immediately thinks of short- and medium-term actions that can have an impact on people's lives. It has been so in the preservation of the memory of people and the spaces in which they were segregated. It is necessary that these heritage sites and the painful, sensitive memories associated with them are preserved for history. The hygienist policy of cleansing society and the devastating impact on those swept up in this policy has to be remembered, so that it never happens again.

This is how the foundation came to hold dozens of meetings to encourage the leaders of the movements of people affected around the world to preserve these places and people's stories. It invited them to visit Hansen's disease museums in Japan, and in this way encouraged them to start projects back in their own countries. Books, autobiographies and biographies, exhibitions and projects for the preservation of oral memory, and many others, are supported by TNF around the world.

With the growth and strengthening of institutions worldwide, the exchange and interaction between them became strategic factors. In this way, in 2019, Mr. Sasakawa, through TNF and the Sasakawa Health Foundation (SHF), stimulated and supported a series of regional meetings that culminated in a Global Forum of People's Organizations on Hansen's Disease, held in Manila, the Philippines, prior to the 20th International Leprosy Congress. The Global Forum brought together approximately eighty people representing entities from eighteen countries to discuss strategies, and was the largest international gathering of its kind. Following the forum, attendees actively participated in the International Leprosy Congress.

If we count participation in regional assemblies leading up to the Global Forum, then the numbers are much higher. The Latin American/Caribbean assembly, held at the Osvaldo Cruz Foundation in Rio de Janeiro, is an example of this. The meeting focused on the third pillar of the WHO's *Global Leprosy Strategy 2016–2020*, which deals with eliminating discrimination and promoting the inclusion of people affected by Hansen's disease, and on the UN Principles and Guidelines on elimination of discrimination against persons affected by leprosy and their family members (both achievements of TNF strategies under Mr. Sasakawa's leadership). The meeting drew a total of 111 participants representing entities and organizations from seven Latin American countries— Bolivia, Brazil, Colombia, Ecuador, Mexico, Paraguay and Peru— as well as members of organizations from the US, Portugal, Germany and Japan, who participated as observers.

On a personal note, around the time of the Global Forum in Manila, I was diagnosed with an aggressive, stage 4, metastatic throat cancer. I postponed the beginning of my treatment as I did not want to stop collaborating with the event and because it was perhaps one of the last opportunities to work closely with

Mr. Sasakawa and so many other people at TNF, for whom I had developed an appreciation and deep respect. Once again, I was encouraged and supported by this leader.

The Global Forum was magnificent, having as one of its outcomes a worldwide campaign and the creation of a logo. It was the first joint campaign supported by TNF/SHF involving people's organizations from different countries. The logo design, which was collectively approved, was accompanied by the campaign slogan: "A Hansen's Disease-Free World with Knowledge and Love". In January 2020, several organizations around the world aligned themselves with a single logo and a single voice around Hansen's disease.

Soon after this action, the COVID-19 pandemic struck and it became necessary for organizations to reinvent themselves, migrate to virtual activities, protect their associates and keep their spirits up in the face of the new challenges that arose. In a very short period, TNF/SHF realized that it was necessary to provide emergency assistance to support persons affected by Hansen's disease, whose vulnerabilities were increasing. In Brazil, hundreds of food baskets, thousands of masks, and hygiene materials were distributed. Lawsuits were filed for the protection of the elderly in the colonies and for them to be given vaccine priority. TNF/SHF and other organizations held meetings and webinars to keep up the fight against Hansen's disease in the context of the pandemic.

As a result of the impact of the pandemic on Hansen's disease services, the number of new cases of Hansen's disease being reported plummeted, and at a higher rate than for other diseases, with the invisibility of the disease reaching levels that could delay its elimination. On the other hand, advances in the field of human rights, the strengthening of organizations of persons affected by Hansen's disease and the empowerment of their leaders have not been reversed.

Once again, the Goodwill Ambassador stepped up and advocated a campaign: "Don't Forget Hansen's Disease". In terms of communication, the easily understood message, combined with an excellent logo and strongly mobilized MORHAN, and via the social networks of other movements, we saw the campaign grow in other countries too. In Brazil, we managed to involve various

117

levels and branches of government, as well as other sectors such as universities, associations, social movements and private institutions. The campaign is still going strong, with several new activities scheduled for the coming months (as of January 2023). Based on a suggestion from the Goodwill Ambassador, TNF/SHF increased its support, including funding, so that organizations could further intensify innovative initiatives to incorporate into the campaign.

I have no doubt as to the historical importance of Mr. Yohei Sasakawa for people affected by Hansen's disease around the world and their organizations. Some of them, including their families, have had their lives damaged by the terrible stigma that Hansen's disease generates. In addition, for those affected and their families, Mr. Sasakawa has been a necessary instrument to promote their dignity throughout the world.

Now, people affected by Hansen's disease are being heard more and have learned to shout. They will not tolerate any setbacks or any loss of rights. But for the foreseeable future, we need Mr. Sasakawa to stay strong in order to amplify the voices and cries of this very vulnerable group.

Had the world known the history of Hansen's disease, and Mr. Sasakawa's paths and strategies to fight the disease and the discrimination, perhaps this knowledge would have helped in the global fight against COVID-19.

5

TOWARDS THE EMPOWERMENT OF
PERSONS WITH LIVED EXPERIENCE OF LEPROSY

Takahiro Nanri

Introduction

Stories of COVID patients and the medical professionals treating them being subjected to discrimination at the height of the coronavirus pandemic have echoes of the experiences of persons affected by leprosy or Hansen's Disease over the years.

Said to be one of humankind's oldest infectious diseases, leprosy was for much of its history a disease without cure. Today, it is treatable with multidrug therapy (MDT) and if the disease is detected and treated promptly, it need not have long-term consequences. But if treatment is delayed, leprosy can result in permanent disability and expose those it affects to social discrimination. Even in the twenty-first century, this discrimination continues. Persons affected by leprosy in various parts of the world find themselves marginalized and their opportunities in life restricted.

But in recent years, they are becoming more vocal about their situation, finding more opportunities to express their views and participate in decision-making that affects them. Ms. Alice Cruz, Special Rapporteur on the Elimination of Discrimination against Persons Affected by Leprosy and Their Family Members, has said, "Participation is key for the long-term elimination of leprosy-related discrimination and for a sustainable inclusion of the affected persons and their family members."[1]

Guidelines for strengthening participation of persons affected by leprosy in leprosy services, published by the World Health Organization (WHO), notes:

> The personal experiences, knowledge and information that persons affected by leprosy have gained through having the disease must be recognised as a valuable asset to enhance the quality of leprosy services. Persons affected by leprosy are the best resource to identify their needs and problems, recommending policy and setting priorities.[2]

Mr. Yohei Sasakawa, the WHO Goodwill Ambassador for Leprosy Elimination as well as the Japanese government's Goodwill Ambassador for the Human Rights of Persons Affected by Leprosy, who also serves as chairman of the Nippon Foundation, can be considered a pioneer in helping to create these trends. For the past almost fifty years, he has spent a great deal of time in fighting leprosy, and has visited more than 100 countries, especially those with a high leprosy burden. In regard to persons affected by leprosy, Mr. Sasakawa said:

> You who have suffered the tyranny of social discrimination are in the best position to correct misconceptions. What you say carries the power of conviction. I know it may be hard to go public because of what you have been through, but the daily discrimination you face as a result of social prejudice is not your fault. It is a disease that afflicts society.[3]

This chapter, as well as reflecting on the specific kinds of support and activities that Mr. Sasakawa has provided for furthering the empowerment of persons affected by leprosy and their family members, also analyzes their significance and ongoing impact.

At the same time, the author considers how the measures of Mr. Sasakawa go beyond the question of leprosy to a higher macro-level awareness, that is, the lessons that we can learn towards "the realization of a society that leaves no one behind", an issue of common concern to all humankind.

1. The main players in the battle against leprosy are the persons affected by it

1–1. Support for the world's first network of persons affected (IDEA)

When the 14th International Leprosy Congress (ILC) was held in August 1993 in Orlando, Florida, USA, there was a workshop on "Consumer and Community Participation in Care and Rehabilitation Programs for Persons with Leprosy", with persons affected by leprosy from six countries, including Japan, the US, Brazil and India, participating for the first time. As Ms. Kay Yamaguchi, former Executive Director of the Sasakawa Memorial Health Foundation (now known as Sasakawa Health Foundation), noted, "This was a landmark event for people involved in leprosy issues, because affected persons from around the world spoke of their existences at a public forum."[4] With the participants in this event as the central players, it was agreed to pursue international alliances of persons affected.

Then, in September 1994, fifty persons affected by leprosy and their supporters from six countries gathered in Petrópolis, Brazil, leading to the establishment of the International Association for Integration, Dignity and Economic Advancement, or IDEA. IDEA serves as a network or platform for persons affected by leprosy around the world, and was a pioneer in this respect. IDEA today has bases of activity in eighteen countries (Angola, Brazil, China, the Democratic Republic of the Congo, Ethiopia, Ghana, India, Kenya, Mozambique, Nepal, Nigeria, Norway, Paraguay, the Philippines, South Korea, Sudan, Taiwan, and the US). However, while some are actively developing their activities, others are not.[5]

Mr. Sasakawa, through the Nippon Foundation, of which he is currently chairman, and through the Sasakawa Health Foundation, a related organization established to tackle leprosy, provided comprehensive support for IDEA's overall activities in its initial period, including financially.[6] Mr. Artur Custódio, former national coordinator of the Movement for the Reintegration of Persons Affected by Hansen's Disease (MORHAN), a Brazilian organization of persons affected by leprosy, writes the following in regard to the role played by Mr. Sasakawa in the process of the establishment and development of IDEA:

> What Mr. Sasakawa, in a visionary way, was already doing at that time, was to provide instruments of empowerment for people with the disease, so that instead of doctors speaking on their behalf, they could exercise their own power of speech and be the protagonists in their struggles to bring about necessary changes to the way the disease was being tackled in their countries and to the policies of the WHO itself.[7]

1–2. Propelling the participation of persons affected in international society

Mr. Sasakawa, following his belief that persons affected by leprosy should themselves play a central role in addressing leprosy issues, also actively supports their participation in international society. For example, in conjunction with the holding of the 60th plenary session of the UN Commission on Human Rights in March 2004, when the Nippon Foundation held a side event on leprosy and human rights for the first time, persons affected by leprosy from India, Brazil and the US were given the opportunity to testify.[8] Also, when Mr. Sasakawa made an oral statement at the 57th session of the UN Sub-Commission on the Promotion and Protection of Human Rights in August 2005, he suddenly suggested to the chair that an opportunity be given for persons affected by leprosy to speak, and four such persons, from India, Nepal and Ghana, were able to speak of their own experiences at the Sub-Commission's session.

Subsequently, after the UN Human Rights Council (established in 2006) adopted in 2008 a Resolution on Elimination of Discrimination against Persons Affected by Leprosy and Their Family

Members, an international conference on leprosy and human rights was held at the UN European Headquarters in January 2009. Mr. Sasakawa exerted efforts to provide an opportunity for persons affected by leprosy from the Philippines, India and Brazil, to speak at this conference.[9]

In 2010, the UN General Assembly unanimously adopted the same resolution and accompanying Principles and Guidelines for the Elimination of Discrimination against Persons Affected by Leprosy and Their Family Members (P&G). Following this, between 2012 and 2015 the Nippon Foundation organized regional symposiums on leprosy and human rights. These were held in Brazil, India, Ethiopia, Morocco and Switzerland, and persons affected from around the globe not only took part, but also played a central role. Moreover, from 2006, in conjunction with World Leprosy Day each January, Mr. Sasakawa began issuing an annual Global Appeal to end stigma and discrimination against persons affected by leprosy.[10]

Supported by different influential individuals and organizations each year, the Global Appeal is designed to raise awareness and promote accurate knowledge and understanding of leprosy. Those who have endorsed the appeal to date include Nobel Peace Prize recipients, leaders of persons affected by leprosy, heads of multi-national corporations and universities, the World Medical Association, the International Bar Association, the International Council of Nurses, the Inter-Parliamentary Union, the International Paralympic Committee, and so on, helping to spread its message far and wide.

Normally at the Global Appeal ceremony, in addition to representatives of the supporting organizations, VIPs of the host country (such as presidents, prime ministers and ministers) give speeches as the main guests. However, Mr. Sasakawa has always invited representatives of persons affected to the venues and provided them with opportunities to speak that are equal to those of the prestigious guests.

When the 10th Global Appeal was held in Tokyo in 2015, about thirty persons affected by leprosy from nine countries took part in the launch ceremony, along with then Prime Minister Shinzo Abe and his wife, and several of them later met with Japan's Emperor and Empress at the Imperial Palace. In June 2016, when the Nippon Foundation co-hosted an international conference at the Vatican titled "Towards Holistic Care for People with Hansen's Disease, Respectful of their Dignity", the approximately 250 participants in the conference included religious leaders, medical practitioners and representatives of international organizations and NGOs from forty-five countries. On that occasion too, Mr. Sasakawa invited around forty persons affected from thirteen countries, and supported their playing a central role in the conference. In January 2023, the Nippon Foundation and Sasakawa Health Foundation, in collaboration with the Dicastery for Promoting Integral Human Development, co-hosted a second international conference at the Vatican on Hansen's disease, with the theme "Leave No One Behind".

1–3. Activities in India

India, which sees the most cases of leprosy, is one of the countries on which Mr. Sasakawa has focused considerable attention. He has travelled to India some sixty times and has visited most of the states in the country. Below, the author discusses the ways in which Mr. Sasakawa has contributed to the empowerment of persons affected by the disease.

(i) The establishment of APAL

Dr. P.K. Gopal, one of the founding members of the above-mentioned IDEA, established IDEA India in 1997. Since 1998, through the Sasakawa Health Foundation, Mr. Sasakawa has supported activities related to this group such as workshops on capacity strengthening, support for education and income generation, and the strengthening of networks of persons affected.

Further, with support from the Nippon Foundation, a survey of leprosy colonies across India was conducted, starting in 2005, with Dr. Gopal playing a leading role. As a result, it became clear that about 750 colonies existed, that residents had a low standard of living, and that many were unable to find regular work and forced to survive by begging.[11] Meanwhile, in December 2005 Mr. Sasakawa held a national conference in which persons affected by leprosy who lived in the colonies participated. In addition to approximately 600 persons affected by leprosy from colonies throughout India, high-level officials such as the minister of social justice and empowerment, and representatives of NGOs, also participated in the conference.

As well as the adoption of the Delhi Declaration of Dignity, which consisted of fourteen recommendations including ensuring that individuals affected by leprosy are not discriminated against in any way in their daily life, and encouraging governments to actively prevent violations of the basic human rights of persons affected, the conference also resulted in the establishment of the National Forum for the Empowerment of People Affected by Leprosy, a networking organization of colony residents that later changed its name to the Association of People Affected by Leprosy, or APAL.

An elderly female participant from Haryana state, with deep emotion expressed her feelings on being able to take part in this conference, as follows: "I did not get the bag and shawl that were given to all delegates, as I was late arriving, but what I got today was something I never got in the last 30 years since I had leprosy: respect and dignity."[12]

Mr. Sasakawa, through the Nippon Foundation and the Sasakawa Health Foundation, has consistently supported APAL since its establishment. APAL aims to improve the social standing of and restore the dignity of persons affected by leprosy, and carries out activities including: 1) network building and empowerment of persons affected; 2) improvement of the living environment in the colonies; and 3) promotion of education and employment opportunities for persons affected by leprosy and their children. Currently, APAL has networks in sixteen states, and is proactively submitting policy proposals to governments and local bodies at the national, state and district levels, to enable persons affected by the disease living in colonies to be able to receive appropriate social services.[13]

One of the noteworthy fruits of APAL's activities was the establishment of a special pension system for persons affected by leprosy. In Report No. 131 of 24 October 2008, India's Rajya Sabha Committee on Petitions flagged nineteen issues to be addressed to improve the situation of persons affected by leprosy. One of these was the proposal that, in order for persons affected by leprosy "to lead an honourable life and not to depend on begging", a monthly stipend of 2,000 rupees should be paid to them as a special pension.[14]

Currently, this special pension specifically for persons affected by leprosy is being paid or considered in at least the Delhi metropolitan area, as well as in the states of Haryana, Bihar, Uttarakhand, Tamil Nadu, Maharashtra, Uttar Pradesh, Madhya Pradesh, Andhra Pradesh, Chhattisgarh and Odisha.[15] Concerning the establishment of these special pensions, it should be noted that Mr. Sasakawa actively encouraged and contributed to efforts by APAL to lobby the authorities in a number of states, helping to make them a reality.

For example, in April 2010, on his visit to the state of Bihar, Mr. Sasakawa met with VIPs such as the state minister of public health. On that occasion, Mr. Sasakawa requested the state authorities to give permission for APAL to take part in these meetings, thus providing them with opportunities to directly address the state minister of public health and others. The APAL representatives, as well as seeking improvement in the living conditions of colony residents, also requested the establishment of a special pension system for those living with serious disabilities resulting from leprosy. To give due consideration to this request, the state authorities asked APAL to provide within two weeks a list of the residents who would be eligible to receive the special pension.

Mr. Sasakawa immediately decided to provide support to cover the cost of the APAL survey, and in fifteen days APAL prepared a list of 997 households in sixty-three colonies within the state. One month later, Mr. Sasakawa revisited the state and, in addition to the minister of public health that he had met before, also had a meeting with the vice governor of the state. Along with APAL, he once again requested the establishment of the special pension system, and was able to succeed in extracting a positive response from the vice premier. In 2012 the state of Bihar established this special pension system: currently, a special stipend of 1,800 rupees is paid monthly.

In the same way, when Mr. Sasakawa visited the state of Uttar Pradesh in October 2013 along with APAL leaders, he met the state governor, the state minister of public health and the state under-secretary of social welfare, requested the establishment of a special pension system in this state, and received a positive response. When Mr. Sasakawa revisited the same state in November 2014 along with APAL, he had a discussion with the state's chief minister, who committed on the spot to the establishment of a special pension system. From the following year, the state decided to pay a monthly stipend of 2,500 rupees (which was subsequently increased to 3,000 rupees). Later, Mr. Sasakawa toured other states such as Chhattisgarh (2017), Odisha (2017), and Andhra Pradesh (2019), where, along with APAL staff, he had discussions with persons in power such as state premiers, health ministers and social welfare ministers, thus contributing to the establishment of a special pension system in those states as well. In these ways, Mr. Sasakawa thoroughly demonstrated his role as an advocate for persons affected by leprosy.

The fact that a special pension system for persons affected by leprosy has been established has clearly contributed to an improvement in the quality of life of persons affected by leprosy who suffer from serious disabilities and so find it difficult to make a living by any means other than begging. In order for this system to be implemented by states, Mr. Sasakawa made sure that whenever he met with high-ranking officials, he provided an opportunity for persons affected to be present and lobby the officials directly. For example, when he met with Indian Prime Minister Narendra Modi in November 2014, Mr. Sasakawa also created an opportunity for APAL members to be present.

The tactic he adopted was to provide opportunities for key officials to listen directly to the voices of the parties concerned and thereby increase the likelihood of policies being implemented. Furthermore, the actions of Mr. Sasakawa brought about greater benefits to persons affected. Through Mr. Sasakawa's efforts, APAL members were able to participate in meetings with various dignitaries, and through this experience they gained confidence and self-respect and have gone on to undertake advocacy around India.

Mr. Vagavathali Narsappa, the former president of APAL, made the following remarks in regard to the role that has been played by Mr. Sasakawa:

> Mr. Sasakawa has been a supporter of APAL over many years, and for us affected persons, he is a colleague who shares the same memories and further has a teacher-like existence. I have never felt like this in relation to anyone else involved in any other donor organization. Mr. Sasakawa, in order to bring about change, kindly thought of the idea that we should stand up and that we "must continue knocking on doors". In other words, even if government parties did not listen to our claims, it was essential to have great patience and to continue to make our claims numerous times.

> As one example of this, Mr. Sasakawa joined us in achieving the establishment of special pension systems in the states of Bihar and Uttar Pradesh. This exerted a strong influence on improving the lifestyle level of affected persons. Also, APAL staff learned many things from Mr. Sasakawa's achievements in these two states and thereafter began similar approaches in other states ourselves, and achieved the establishment of the same kinds of pension systems. Mr. Sasakawa is a person who has unceasingly provided us with inspiration in regard to the direction we should follow. The things we have learned from Mr. Sasakawa can definitely not be calculated in terms such as money.[16]

(ii) The establishment of S-ILF

As a result of the above-mentioned nationwide colony survey, Mr. Sasakawa, determining that more organized and large-scale assistance was needed to support the self-dependence of persons affected living in the colonies, established the Sasakawa-India Leprosy Foundation (S-ILF) in November 2006. In order to assist persons affected by leprosy and their family members who were residents of the approximately 750 colonies in India, S-ILF undertook livelihood projects to promote economic self-reliance utilizing microcredit; support for education through the provision of scholarships for persons affected by leprosy and their children; and occupational training.

In regard to his objective in establishing S-ILF, Mr. Sasakawa said: "It is to rid India of begging undertaken by persons affected by leprosy." Concerning the realization of this dream, Mr. Sasakawa himself, and his good friend Mr. Murlidhar Devidas Amte (Baba Amte), made the following comparison with the Anandvan community, where persons affected by leprosy were then living. At Anandvan, a self-sufficient community established in 1949, residents carried out a wide range of productive activities:

> The objectives of S-ILF, which I launched in India, are to remove the social prejudice and discrimination against persons affected by leprosy, support their economic independence, and achieve their integration to society. Moreover, Anandvan has proved that such economic independence is possible, and provided many hints and lessons for S-ILF in its future activities.[17]

The author would also like to mention the Dalai Lama–Sasakawa Scholarship project that was launched by Mr. Sasakawa with the cooperation of His Holiness the 14th Dalai Lama, who likewise is passionate about the resolution of leprosy issues, and in the past has met with Mr. Sasakawa several times. According to Mr. Sasakawa, one day the following conversation took place between them.

First, when Mr. Sasakawa spoke of his dream to reduce to zero the number of people living in leprosy colonies who survive by begging, the Dalai Lama replied: "It would be impossible to realize that." In response, Mr. Sasakawa said, "The only way to discover if it is impossible or not is to try." In reply, the Dalai Lama agreed, saying: "Yes, it is as you say."[18]

Perhaps because he remembered this conversation, when the two of them visited a leprosy colony in Delhi together in March 2014, the Dalai Lama offered to donate the royalties from the sales of his books to persons affected by leprosy. As a result, a scholarship fund project to provide support for residents of the colonies to advance to institutes of higher education was launched. Currently, as of December 2022, scholarships are being paid to 178 residents of colonies in eleven states of India through this scholarship fund system.[19]

Mr. Sasakawa, in order to advance other projects to improve the quality of life of persons affected and for the streamlining of appropriate legal systems, determined that cooperation with parliamentarians was required, and in October 2012 launched the Forum of Parliamentarians to Free India of Leprosy. Incidentally, S-ILF serves as the administration office for both the above-mentioned scholarship fund project and this alliance.

1–4. Activities in Brazil

In Brazil, which reports the world's second highest number of annual new cases of leprosy, Mr. Sasakawa has provided support to MORHAN, a nationwide movement for the reintegration of persons affected by leprosy. The central members of MORHAN are residents of former leprosy hospital-colonies. The organization was established in 1981 with the objectives of achieving the elimination of discrimination against persons affected by Hansen's disease and their family members, restoring their dignity, reintegrating them into society and improving public health services.

As of March 2022, MORHAN carries out its activities through seventy-two branches in twenty-three states, and has 2,524 volunteer members.[20] Included among the volunteers are not only affected persons, but also people from a wide range of sectors, such as medical practitioners, lawyers, researchers and pro bono workers. In addition to providing care for affected persons, providing information about leprosy, making policy proposals and conducting advocacy and awareness-raising, MORHAN's wide-ranging activities also extend to the management and administration of a former hospital-colony in Rio de Janeiro state.

MORHAN is arguably the most dynamic organization of persons affected in the world and a leader at the global level. Mr. Sasakawa has supported its activities both openly and in the background. For example, Mr. Sasakawa, through the Nippon Foundation, has since 2004 been supporting MORHAN's nationwide TELEHANSEN project. This is an information hotline staffed by MORHAN volunteers who answer questions about leprosy via telephone calls, SNS messages and the Internet.

In particular, for callers who suspect they have leprosy or patients who have been diagnosed with the disease, TELEHANSEN volunteers can provide advice based on their own personal experiences, enabling more nuanced responses. According to the MORHAN office, in the one-year period from June 2018 to May 2019, there was a total of 4,227 enquiries; of these, 998 were via the website and 1,778 via SNS.[21] In regard to the content of these enquiries, in addition to questions about the disease, there were also questions about government compensation and participating in MORHAN as a volunteer, as well as requests from the media for interviews. In this way, MORHAN is fulfilling some functions that government and local bodies do not, while playing an important role in promoting the empowerment of persons affected.

Some of MORHAN's policy proposals have produced some impressive results. The group played an essential role in the process of achieving the enactment of Law 11,520 in 2007, which implemented financial compensation for residents of former hospital-colonies. As of February 2022, 9,039 people have received compensation.[22] MORHAN is currently aiming for the enactment of laws to provide compensation to persons born in hospital-colonies who were forcibly separated from their parents and sent to orphanages, or given up for adoption, because their parents had leprosy.

Further, some MORHAN representatives participate in the health councils of central government and various states, and are involved in the process of drafting and implementing public health measures at the national and state levels. According to Mr. Artur Custódio, former national coordinator of MORHAN, the National Health Council, as an advisory body to the Ministry of Health, has the function of supervising the drafting and implementation of policies; of its forty-eight members, half are representatives of citizens' groups. There are also councils at the state level that possess the same types of functions. MORHAN, by proactively utilizing these opportunities, is contributing to the drafting and implementation of leprosy-related policies.

In the same way as he had done in India, Mr. Sasakawa, when holding discussions with those in powerful positions in his capacity as WHO Goodwill Ambassador for Leprosy Elimination, set up opportunities for members of MORHAN to participate and speak directly with the VIPs. For example, when he visited Brazil in December 2008, Mr. Sasakawa met then President Luiz Inácio Lula da Silva accompanied by seven members of MORHAN. Perhaps influenced by the opportunity to hear directly from persons affected themselves, the federal government subsequently added leprosy issues as a topic for priority treatment by local government bodies.

In December 2013, when Mr. Sasakawa met with Ms. Maria do Rosário Nunes, head of the Secretariat for Human Rights of the Presidency of the Federal Republic of Brazil, forty persons affected by leprosy and their family members also took part, discussing the above-mentioned issue of support for children born to parents with leprosy, and the Secretary expressed her intent to support such measures.

Moreover, when Mr. Sasakawa visited Brazil in July 2019, he had a meeting with the then President Jair Bolsonaro that two members of MORHAN also attended. Partway through the meeting, at the president's suggestion, they directly appealed to the people of Brazil about the importance of tackling leprosy issues via Facebook Live, with the president, Mr. Sasakawa and a MORHAN representative participating. On the same visit to Brazil, when Mr. Sasakawa travelled to the states of Pará and Maranhão, he was always accompanied by MORHAN representatives in discussions with state governors and high-level state officials.

In his chapter in this book, Mr. Custódio has made the following comments in regard to the role played by Mr. Sasakawa:

> His harmony with the basic needs of people with the disease and his enterprising and humanitarian outlook marked the beginning of a partnership of brothers that would last until today.

> I cannot begin to count how many times Mr. Sasakawa has been present at activities organized by MORHAN. ... he firmly defended the inclusion of MORHAN in decision-making spaces, even if he sometimes put himself in difficult situations from a diplomatic standpoint.

> I have no doubt as to the historical importance of Mr. Yohei Sasakawa for people affected by Hansen's disease around the world and their organizations.[23]

1–5. Activities in Indonesia

In Indonesia, the country with the third highest number of leprosy cases, the focus of Mr. Sasakawa's support is PerMaTa, an

Indonesian organization of persons affected by leprosy. After PerMaTa was established in 2007, the Sasakawa Health Foundation supported it consistently. As of late January 2021, PerMaTa has twenty-nine branches in four provinces (South Sulawesi, East Nusa Tenggara, East Java and South Sumatra) and about 2,100 affiliated members.[24]

Like MORHAN, PerMaTa also follows the principle of having its members or volunteer base participate in all its activities. However, unlike MORHAN, all of PerMaTa's membership is composed of persons affected by leprosy. Compared to APAL and MORHAN, PerMaTa operates on a small scale and not on a nation-wide basis. However, as a group organized by persons affected themselves, it is the largest in Indonesia, and can be expected to develop further in the future. A feature of PerMaTa's activities is that psychological care and advice on medical matters is given directly to leprosy patients by members based on their own experi-ence. Since care of leprosy patients is not only about the disease itself but also about mental health issues, it is important that PerMaTa members, who are themselves affected by the disease, should be directly involved. In recent years, there is growing awareness of the value of the role played by PerMaTa. For exam-ple, in 2018 it was agreed that the Ministry of Health and PerMaTa would jointly carry out awareness raising activities in provinces with a high incidence of leprosy.[25]

As well as the above, PerMaTa also implements other activities such as empowerment of its members, support for economic inde-pendence and education, and leadership training. Further, since PerMaTa does not operate nationwide, the group has utilized the strategy of joining with movements of persons with disabilities so as to be involved in a wide range of policy proposals and educa-tional activities.

One positive result of the above is the establishment of the Multi-Stakeholder Forum, for the purpose of comprehensive dis-cussion on overall issues related to persons with disabilities, includ-ing those with leprosy-related disabilities, at the state level. The members of this forum discuss together in a comprehensive fashion a wide range of issues related to disability, with participants including relevant government departments (such as public health, social security and education) and organizations, international NGOs and other interested persons. By October 2018, similar types of forum had also been launched in three other provinces: East Java, South Sulawesi and East Nusa Tenggara.

In the same way as he had done in India and Brazil, Mr. Sasakawa provided opportunities for persons connected with PerMaTa to participate in his meetings with top-ranking officials and express their views in person. For example, in June 2009, Mr. Sasakawa, along with the Association of Southeast Asian Nations (ASEAN) Secretariat, hosted a ceremony in Jakarta to launch a project on Leprosy and Human Dignity. This was attended by approximately 160 people, including government and media representatives, as well as Mr. Surin Pitsuwan, the secretary-general of ASEAN (and former foreign minister of Thailand) and other VIPs, and the chairman of PerMaTa was also an important participant.

When, in December 2016, Mr. Sasakawa had a meeting with the minister of health Professor Nila Moeloek, he expressed his hope that the government would involve PerMaTa in its activities against leprosy. In November 2017, PerMaTa representatives also participated on-site when Mr. Sasakawa had meetings with Vice President Jusuf Kalla and Mr. Anies Baswedan, governor of Jakarta. Furthermore, from 2017 to 2018, when Mr. Sasakawa made visits to leprosy-endemic provinces including North Sulawesi, Gorontalo, South Sulawesi, Central Sulawesi, North Maluku and Maluku, where he held meetings with core state, district and city government figures, PerMaTa members attended almost all the meetings.

Mr. Sasakawa considered it important in Indonesia to take part in television and radio talk shows, and to carry out awareness raising activities along with PerMaTa staff. In recent years, Indonesian media channels that have featured Mr. Sasakawa include: Radio Republik Indonesia, TVRI Gorontalo (November 2017, Gorontalo State); TVRI Makassar, Gamasi 105.9 FM (March 2018, South Sulawesi State); TVRI Palu, Radio Republik Indonesia (March 2018, Central Sulawesi State); and TVRI Maluku, Radio Republik Indonesia (North Maluku Province, October 2018). He believed that these activities were not only for awareness raising purposes, but also provided opportunities for PerMaTa members to proactively express their personal views through public media, and thus made a major contribution to increasing their confidence and reducing their self-stigma.[26]

Mr. Al Kadri, the current chairman of PerMaTa and a leader of its South Sulawesi branch, made the following remarks in regard to Mr. Sasakawa:

> Mr. Sasakawa is very instrumental in establishing and supporting PerMaTa, so that many people affected by leprosy are empowered and able to socialize like me. By involving us in his visits to meet with officials, such as regents, governors and even vice presidents, it certainly raises our dignity. Involving us to talk on TV and radio made our confidence increase and of course it became a source of pride for us. From this talk show, many of my family in the village were proud of me because, even though I had had leprosy and never went to school, I could talk on TV with foreigners and the government.[27]

1–6. Activities in Ethiopia and elsewhere

Mr. Sasakawa's activities to support persons affected in other countries are outlined below. In Ethiopia, Mr. Sasakawa has provided support to the Ethiopian National Association of Persons Affected by Leprosy (ENAPAL), an organization established in 1996 that currently has seventy-three branches across seven of Ethiopia's eleven zones and about 20,000 members.[28] As elsewhere, Mr. Sasakawa has made a point of involving leaders of persons affected by leprosy in his meetings with top officials. For example, when he visited the country in February 2006 and met with Prime Minister Meles Zenawi, representatives of ENAPAL were present and scenes from the event were given major coverage in the *Ethiopian Herald* newspaper the following day.

In the same way, in July 2010 and April 2015 when he met with the minister of health, ENAPAL representatives also participated. And when the third in the series of regional symposiums on leprosy and human rights was held in Addis Ababa in September 2013, along with Prime Minister Hailemariam Desalegn and the health minister Keseteberhan Admasu, ENAPAL representatives took part as central participants. Mr. Sasakawa has also contributed to strengthening the organizational base of ENAPAL through the financial support of the Sasakawa Health Foundation. When Mr. Sasakawa visited Ethiopia in July 2018, he learned that ENAPAL had received a plot of land from the government on which to build a new headquarters. ENAPAL's plan was to rent out space in the building to generate income and put it on a path to self-sustainability. On hearing this, Mr. Sasakawa agreed, following a feasibility study, to fund construction of the new building.

Work on the project was completed in September 2022 and a grand opening ceremony was held in the presence of Mr. Sasakawa, as well as Ethiopia's minister of women and social affairs, minister of health and the WHO Country Representative to Ethiopia. The building is currently home to a private school corporation that runs from a kindergarten through to high school. Through the administering of this building, if ENAPAL is able to secure a steady source of income and conduct sustainable business operations, it could become a model to consider for other organizations of persons affected by leprosy.

Mr. Tesfaye Tadesse, former managing director of ENAPAL, made the following remarks in regard to Mr. Sasakawa:

> Mr. Yohei Sasakawa was one of the founding fathers of ENAPAL from the inception. Despite his relatively advanced age he is the sole person who went to remote leprosy villages in Ethiopia where no one visited. Many members of ENAPAL have got educational opportunities and socio-economic support that help them to break the vicious circle of poverty and discrimination. With the help of the Goodwill Ambassador, the ENAPAL chairperson was able to enter the offices of Prime Minister Meles Zenawi and the minister of health. With all walks of support, ENAPAL regional and local associations became able to advocate for the rights of their members. The history of discrimination and stigma upon Persons Affected by Leprosy is reversed constructively through the ENAPAL HQ income-generating and training center supported by SHF in the center of Addis Ababa. The building is not only income-generating, it is emblematic and a means of organizational sustainability that helps ENAPAL to exist independently.[29]

There are many other examples of Mr. Sasakawa's beneficial activities working through the Sasakawa Health Foundation. Handa Rehabilitation and Welfare Association (HANDA) was the first grassroots NGO to receive permission to directly support persons affected by leprosy in China, providing support to around 3,000 people. Established in 1996 in Guangdong Province, HANDA has to date provided services to 217 leprosy recovery villages in fourteen provinces, mainly working in Guangdong, Guangxi and Yunnan. The SHF has also provided support to other organizations, including: the Coalition of Leprosy Advocates in the Philippines, or CLAP (established in 2012), a network of persons affected and supporters, comprising an affiliation of nineteen NGOs focusing on persons affected by leprosy within the Philippines; Felehansen (established in 2014), a group comprising nine organizations of persons affected in Colombia; and the Myanmar Association of People Affected by Leprosy (MAPAL, established in 2014). In addition, through the Nippon Foundation/Sasakawa Health Foundation, Mr. Sasakawa has also supported IDEA Nepal (established in 1998), a member of the previously mentioned IDEA; and IDEA Ghana (established in 2003).

In total, the support that Mr. Sasakawa has provided up to now through the two foundations has assisted thirty-seven groups of persons affected by leprosy in twenty-two countries, and amounts to 1.54 billion yen (see Table 5 for the list of groups supported by the two foundations). Moreover, in December 2019, the two foundations supported the first ever nationwide conference for persons affected by leprosy in Bangladesh, after Mr. Sasakawa proposed the idea to Prime Minister Sheikh Hasina earlier in the year, and supported the launching of a nationwide organization of persons affected by leprosy there.

Mr. Amar Timalsina, who has served as the long-time representative of IDEA Nepal, has made the following remarks:

> Mr. Sasakawa has made selfless, tireless and immense contributions to empower the global community of persons who have experienced Hansen's disease/leprosy. Because of his presence, we could feel like we have always been supported by our guardian. Mr. Sasakawa's contribution in the field of leprosy is unprecedented.[30]

In the same vein, Mr. Kofi Nyarko, president of IDEA Ghana, has said:

> You can't talk about persons affected by Hansen's disease and their empowerment without mentioning Mr. Sasakawa. Even the way he humbles himself every time he visits Hansen's disease settlements and interacts with the persons affected gives us a lot of hope in life. Affected people always admire his contribution to our society and we all pray that he will live a long life so that he achieves all his dreams.[31]

Considering that Mr. Amar and Mr. Kofi have both been driving forces behind movements of persons affected by leprosy around the world, it is no exaggeration to say that their comments reflect the views of many other persons affected as well.

1–7. Holding the Global Forum

One of the highlights of Mr. Sasakawa's activities in support of persons affected was the Global Forum of People's Organizations on Hansen's Disease, which was held from 7 to 10 September 2019 under the auspices of the Nippon Foundation and the Sasakawa Health Foundation, in Manila, the Philippines. About eighty representatives of groups of persons affected in twenty-three countries participated in the Global Forum, whose objectives were: 1) to broadly disseminate the voices of persons affected by leprosy at the 20th International Leprosy Congress meeting that was held immediately after the Global Forum, and 2) to exchange information and share views among those taking part in order to contribute to the strengthening of each of the participating organizations.

The conference focused on three main themes: human rights, the sustainability of organizations, and the participation of persons affected by leprosy in decisions that affected their lives.[32] One of the results of the meeting was the adoption of the Conclusions and Recommendations based on the agreement of all participants (the Manila Declaration). An outline of this Declaration is below:[33]

- Full and impactful participation of People's Organizations in policy-making processes concerning Hansen's disease must be assured.

- People's Organizations must actively advocate for quality Hansen's disease services within an integrated health structure and system and through their committed participation help ensure the sustainability of the Hansen's disease program.
- People's Organizations should strengthen existing networks and create truly functioning regional and global networks.
- Governments and other partners should be open and willing to fund projects that address the sustainability of People's Organizations in recognition of the contribution these organizations can make.

Given that the Global Forum was held immediately prior to the 20th International Leprosy Congress where all the different stakeholders in leprosy gathered, and that persons affected from around the world could speak with a united voice, it had a big impact in terms of raising awareness among Congress delegates of the existence of persons affected and the issues they face.

Further, the Nippon Foundation and the Sasakawa Health Foundation held a 2nd Global Forum in Hyderabad, India, prior to the 21st International Leprosy Congress in November 2022. The Forum was a hybrid in-person and online event, with approximately 100 people representing people's organizations from twenty-one countries taking part, and new Conclusions and Recommendations were adopted.[34]

Mr. Sasakawa has also been actively supporting groups of persons affected during the COVID-19 pandemic. With support from the Nippon Foundation, in November 2020 the Sasakawa Health Foundation established a grant programme for organizations of persons affected by leprosy and has provided financial help totalling approximately 50 million yen to twenty-two groups from eighteen countries.

This programme carried out assistance in three fields: responses to the direct needs of persons affected, advocacy, and information dissemination. Unlike emergency assistance measures supported by other international NGOs, these projects do not limit persons affected solely to the role of aid recipients, but rather by positioning them as major contributing actors in COVID relief projects; in this way the projects are intended to raise their awareness and strengthen their capacity, and thus reduce self-stigma.

2. What is the significance of the activities of Mr. Sasakawa?

2–1. Cultivating the trend of focusing on persons affected

As noted above, Mr. Sasakawa has continued to support persons affected by leprosy in a variety of ways, as a result of which two trends have emerged.

First, in many places all over the globe, organizations of persons affected have been established, of varying sizes and forms. As mentioned earlier, the Sasakawa Health Foundation and the Nippon Foundation are supporting thirty-seven groups of persons affected in twenty-two countries. According to a survey conducted by Ms. Paula Brandao, a volunteer of MORHAN, the Brazilian organization of persons affected, currently forty-nine groups of persons affected in twenty-seven countries have been established that can be confirmed. If we added the self-help groups that exist in various places around the world, although they may not be formally organized, the total number would be enormous.

At the aforementioned Global Forum in Manila, there were discussions on the promotion of participation by persons affected by leprosy, and their empowerment, and in the Manila Declaration finally adopted by the Forum, it was agreed that networks of persons affected on the global level should be strengthened. Given the progress made around the world in organizing persons affected by leprosy since the founding of IDEA in 1994, it is impossible to think of this happening without the contribution of Mr. Sasakawa.

Second, recognition of the importance of having policies that centre on persons affected, in a wide range of political measures and programmes, is spreading. The Principles and Guidelines for the Elimination of Leprosy Discrimination (P&G) adopted by the United Nations General Assembly in 2010 note:

> In the development and implementation of legislation and policies and in other decision-making processes concerning issues relating

to persons affected by leprosy and their family members, States should consult closely with and actively involve persons affected by leprosy and their family members, individually or through their respective local and national organizations.[35]

The WHO, which plays a central role in overseeing global leprosy strategy, has now made it obligatory to consider issues of discrimination and stigma in measures to address leprosy. For example, as noted earlier, in 2011 the WHO established *Guidelines for Strengthening Participation of Persons Affected by Leprosy in Leprosy Services*, and recommended the participation of persons affected at every stage of leprosy services. Further, from 2006, the Global Leprosy Programme (GLP), which oversees the WHO's leprosy strategy, has set global strategies related to leprosy measures every five years. In the GLP's *Global Leprosy Strategy 2016–2020: Accelerating towards a leprosy-free world*, fully eliminating stigma and discrimination related to leprosy is one of the four parts of its vision of a leprosy-free world, and the strategy recommends that collaboration with persons affected takes place in addressing both the medical and social aspects of each country's leprosy policies.[36]

This policy is also followed in the *Towards Zero Leprosy: Global Leprosy (Hansen's Disease) Strategy 2021–2030*, released in 2021.[37] We can see that in order for countries to determine policies based on the GLP strategies, it is gradually becoming mainstream to have policies that advance collaboration with persons affected in national leprosy measures.

2–2. The uniqueness of the tactics employed by Mr. Sasakawa

As described in this chapter, based on his view that "the main players in the fight against leprosy are the affected persons themselves", Mr. Sasakawa has furthered the empowerment of persons affected by leprosy through his own unique strategies.

According to the United Nations, empowerment is "the process of enabling people to increase control over their lives, to gain control over the factors and decisions that shape their lives, to increase their resources and qualities and to build capacities to gain access, partners, networks, a voice, in order to gain control".[38] In other words, so that the path that should be taken by persons affected by leprosy can be decided by the persons themselves, Mr. Sasakawa first took the lead by establishing a wide range of opportunities, and then promoting the participation of persons affected on those occasions. For example, these might include setting up venues for persons affected to express their views and give speeches at international conferences, or enabling the participation of persons affected in meetings with persons holding the highest level of responsibility at the state or national level.

Persons affected by leprosy who as a result of long-standing discrimination from society suffered from self-stigma and tended to become withdrawn or introverted, through expressing their own ideas and opinions in situations like this, and through making proposals related to specific government policies or measures, little by little gained confidence and experience. Moreover, many of the persons affected who participated in these events were able to recover their self-respect. Subsequently, they began to express their thoughts at a wide range of venues, and this movement has spread throughout the globe. Mr. Sasakawa kept abreast of these trends and provided support for the development of organizations of persons affected by leprosy through the Nippon Foundation and the Sasakawa Health Foundation, and through his personal interaction with their leaders. In other words, the empowerment implemented by Mr. Sasakawa consisted of restoring the dignity of persons affected and helping them to organize.

Up until the present, those involved in dealing with leprosy issues have addressed the empowerment of persons affected in a variety of ways, such as by implementing grassroots training and educational activities. However, there is no example of a more bold, dynamic and clear-cut policy-based tactic than that employed by Mr. Sasakawa.

2–3. What is meant by the versatility of a more global approach?

Next, the author would like to discuss how the measures taken by Mr. Sasakawa have gone beyond the framework of leprosy issues, and their versatility at a more global level. First, concerning the measures carried out by Mr. Sasakawa related to empowerment of persons affected, there is the possibility that these could be slotted within existing frameworks such as "health and human rights" or "infectious diseases and human rights". For example, leprosy is not the only neglected tropical disease (NTD) that can leave lingering disabilities that cause stigma and discrimination.

However, efforts to organize and empower persons affected by NTDs as a whole have not gone as far as efforts to organize and empower persons affected by leprosy, with persons affected by NTDs generally still positioned as recipients of aid, as were persons affected by leprosy around the time Mr. Sasakawa began his efforts to assist them.

While it is not easy to immediately implement what Mr. Sasakawa has done, the approach promoted by him of creating opportunities for persons affected to participate in various ways, while at the same time providing parallel support to help them become more organized, can be effective.

Second, from a broader perspective, that of aiming for the realization of "a society where no one gets left behind" as put forth in the UN's Sustainable Development Goals (SDGs), we have many things to learn from Mr. Sasakawa's measures. For example, in order to achieve the SDGs, it is essential to help the socially vulnerable find their feet. Hence, the support provided to persons affected by leprosy undertaken by Mr. Sasakawa provides us with concrete models as to how we should relate to persons affected and the actions we should take.

In these ways, the tactics Mr. Sasakawa has developed and the activities he has carried out in support of persons affected by leprosy transcend leprosy. In addressing common concerns that all human beings face, they provide us with many lessons.

3. In conclusion

The author has been fortunate to have had many opportunities to accompany Mr. Sasakawa and participate in numerous activities mentioned in this article. During these, something the author found surprising was the stance of Mr. Sasakawa when attending meetings with highly placed persons. As remarked earlier, Mr. Sasakawa established a wide range of opportunities in which persons affected by leprosy could participate. On such occasions, Mr. Sasakawa's considered approach was evident.

Specifically, he would always take a step back and never forgot to put forward the persons affected. At the start of many meetings Mr. Sasakawa would summarize the purpose and desired outcome, and then he would usually say something along the following lines: "For more detailed information, please ask the affected persons who are present, directly." This stance was unchanging whether the other party was a mere official, or whether he or she was the president or prime minister of the country.

On one occasion, Mr. Sasakawa said the following to the author:

> It's not that I personally have the objective of meeting a president or prime minister. But through discussions with these kinds of people, I anticipate that progress will be made on resolving issues, such as policies being made or new budget measures being put in place. Moreover, if affected persons can participate at these venues, their words are many times more persuasive than my own.

It is not all that difficult to say that "in the fight against leprosy, the main actors are the persons affected". Nowadays many people mention this. Furthermore, we can glimpse the same kind of expression in a wide range of policy documents. Yet for how many people is this actually the case? One of Mr. Sasakawa's favourite mottos is "Knowledge as action". That is, even if there is knowledge, unless this knowledge is actually put into practice, it is completely meaningless.

In order to eliminate discrimination and stigma against persons affected by leprosy, if there were even a few more people who thought and acted like Mr. Yohei Sasakawa, there is no doubt the current conditions would improve from their present state. The author earnestly hopes that this will happen.

Table 5: The organizations of persons affected by leprosy supported by TNF and SHF (as of March 2022)

Country	Organization	Organization	Period of Support	Amount (JPY thousand)	Supporting organisation
Global	IDEA International	IDEA International	1997–2007 1996–2011	232,741 65,013	TNF SHF
Bangladesh	ALO	Advancing Leprosy and Disadvantaged Peoples Opportunities Society	2020–2021	2,670	SHF
Bangladesh	Bogra Federation	Bogura Zilla Kushtho O Protibondahi Unnayan Shonguthan	2020–2021	6,377	SHF
Brazil	MORHAN	Movement for the Reintegration of Persons Affected by Hansen's Disease	2003–2018	212,563	TNF
Brazil	MORHAN	Movement for the Reintegration of Persons Affected by Hansen's Disease	2004 2006 2012 2019–2021	53,684	SHF
China	HANDA	HANDA Rehabilitation and Welfare Association	1995 1999–2021	220,735	SHF
Colombia	Corsohansen	Corsohansen	2011–2016	16,476	SHF

Colombia	Felehansen	National Federation of People Affected by Leprosy of Colombia	2018	4,472	SHF
Ethiopia	ENAPAL	Ethiopian National Association of Persons Affected by Leprosy	2001–2021	172,714	SHF
Ghana	IDEA Ghana	IDEA Ghana	2004–2005 2008–2013 2017–2018 2021	18,721	SHF
India	APAL	Association of People Affected by Leprosy	2005–2019 2020–2021	140,851 20,413	TNF SHF
India	Atma Swabhiman	Atma Swabhiman	2020–2021	2,998	SHF
India	IDEA India	IDEA India	1998–2014	159,151	SHF
India	National Forum	National Forum—India	2005–2009	14,514	SHF
India	SKNSS	Sahyog Kusth Nivaran Sangh Samiti, Indore	2021	1,545	SHF
India	SKSS	Saksham Kushthanteya Swabhimani Sanstha	2020–2021	2,609	SHF
Indonesia	PerMaTa	Perhimpunan Mandiri Kusta Indonesia	2008–2018 2020–2021	52,430	SHF

Kenya	IDEA Kenya	IDEA REFACO Kenya Foundation	2020	1,028	SHF
Malaysia	—	Sungai Buloh Settlement Council	2017–2018	7,839	SHF
Mozambique	ALEMO	Association of People Affected by Leprosy in Mozambique	2020–2021	1,280	SHF
Mozambique	AMPAL	Associação Moçambicana de Pessoas Atingidas por Lepra	2021	1,247	SHF
Myanmar	MAPAL	Myanmar Association of Persons Affected by Leprosy	2021	2,605	SHF
Nepal	IDEA Nepal	Association for IDEA Nepal	2002 2004–2008 2010 2014 2020–2021	11,392	SHF
Nepal	SHG Federation	Dhanusha, Mahottari, Sarlahi and Sindhuli Self–Help Group Federations	2020–2021	5,308	SHF
Niger	IDEA Niger	Association for Integration, Dignity and Economic Advancement	2020–2021	2,447	SHF
Nigeria	IDEA Nigeria	IDEA Nigeria	2020	1,196	SHF
Nigeria	PHIN	Purple Hope Initiative Nigeria	2020	825	SHF

Country	Abbreviation	Organization	Years	Number	Fund
Philippines	ACHI	Association of Culion Hansenites, Inc.	2003–2005	3,566	SHF
Philippines	CLAP	Coalition of Leprosy Advocates of the Philippines	2009–2010 2013–2018	60,697	SHF
Philippines	IDEA Eversley	IDEA Eversley	2003	491	SHF
Philippines	PGH Hansen's Club	PGH Hansen's Club	2020	321	SHF
Senegal	ASCL/MTN	Association Sénégalaise de Lutte Contre la Lèpre et les Maladies Tropicales Négligées	2020–2021	1,282	SHF
Sierra Leone	NAPAL-SL	National Association of Persons Affected by Leprosy Sierra Leone	2020–2021	1,022	SHF
Tanzania	TLA	Tanzania Leprosy Association	2008–2010	12,601	SHF
Japan	–	Resident Committee, National Sanatorium Kuryu Rakusen-en	2015–2016	600	SHF
Japan	–	Resident Committee, National Sanatorium, Hoshizuka Keiai-en	2020	19,000	SHF
			Total	1,056,806 (586,155) (949,269)	TNF SHF

6

WHY PUBLIC AWARENESS MUST BE PROMOTED

ROLE OF THE WHO GOODWILL AMBASSADOR
FOR LEPROSY ELIMINATION

Tatsuya Tanami

Introduction

Recognizing his strong commitment and leadership in the fight to eliminate leprosy (Hansen's disease), in January 2001 the World Health Organization appointed Yohei Sasakawa as Special Ambassador representing the Global Alliance for the Elimination of Leprosy (GAEL). When this alliance was disbanded in 2003, the name of his position was changed to WHO Goodwill Ambassador for Leprosy Elimination. January 2021 marked the 20th anniversary of his initial appointment as Special Ambassador to the Global Alliance.

Mr. Sasakawa's thoughts regarding the role and responsibilities of the WHO Goodwill Ambassador for Leprosy Elimination were outlined in his first "Ambassador's Newsletter". In his message, he

149

states that the first objective of the Special Ambassador's work is to instill in political leaders of countries where leprosy remains endemic a strong commitment to its elimination, and the second is to have the media call attention to the disease in a way that gives the general public a correct understanding of leprosy. At the same time, he stressed the importance of sharing correct knowledge and information to the non-leprosy community—individuals and organizations working to address social issues not directly related to leprosy—to spread this correct knowledge and information more widely among the general public in the course of their work. He also noted that the ultimate goal of the newsletter was to convey information to a broad audience, stressing the importance of conveying correct knowledge and information regarding leprosy to broader society beyond the leprosy community, from top to bottom, from political leaders to the general public.[1]

The second issue of the newsletter addressed the issue of "From Vertical to Horizontal", citing Myanmar as an example. In Myanmar, the key was to shift from a vertical structure of professional organizations and specialists to a horizontal structure that went beyond leprosy specialists to include general health workers, NGOs and media personalities.[2] This helped to convey the message that leprosy is a curable disease that need not be feared, and led to policies that did not miss opportunities to provide effective and timely medical treatment.

Mr. Sasakawa was concerned that people did not know about leprosy. In his book *Making the Impossible Possible* (2021), he presented various anecdotes. When he visited Uganda in June 2001 and met with President Yoweri Museveni of Uganda, he was very surprised when President Museveni told him that "leprosy was unheard of in his country". The fact was that the president of an African country had not been informed about the situation regarding leprosy.[3] This problem was not limited to Africa, however. Mr. Sasakawa summarized the problem he felt about people "not knowing" as follows:

1) Knowledge and information about leprosy was only being exchanged within leprosy circles.

2) With the number of persons affected by leprosy declining, the disease was no longer a social issue.

3) It was thought of as a problem that no longer existed.

4) Regardless of what people in general society did or did not know about leprosy, they mistakenly understood it to be hereditary, a divine punishment, a dangerous infectious disease, an incurable disease, etc.

5) This lack of knowledge led to fear and prejudice.

6) This lack of knowledge existed in people from government leaders to otherwise well-informed people, the media, the general public and persons affected by leprosy. There were even cases of medical doctors who misunderstood the disease.

Why was it necessary to build awareness to instill a correct understanding around the world?

1) So that infected people would not be afraid to receive diagnosis and treatment, the only way to prevent the disease from spreading.

2) To detect the disease early before physical disabilities develop.

3) So that infected persons could receive compassionate care from their family, community and society.

4) To prevent infected people and their families from being discriminated against.

5) As an effective way to reduce social and medical costs.

6) As an effective way to provide a path to employment for persons affected by leprosy, so they could make a social and economic contribution.

How to cope with the above problems? Mr. Sasakawa came to the following conclusions:

1) The problems of leprosy and resulting discrimination should be seen as current-day problems that are a negative legacy that has burdened humankind throughout history, rather than as a minor social problem or a problem that existed in the past.

2) The media should be used effectively. Various opportunities, including the submission of articles, press conferences, advertising and appearances on radio and television programmes should be used.

3) A correct message about the disease should be disseminated to influential people and organizations.
4) Opportunities should be created for influential people and organizations to participate in activities to eliminate social discrimination.
5) Religious leaders should disseminate a correct message to their followers.
6) An ambassador for leprosy elimination should travel to local areas and use opportunities like press conferences so that local media will report correct information.
7) The United Nations should be approached to pass a human rights resolution and implement and disseminate principles and guidelines.

1. Yohei Sasakawa's activities to promote social awareness

Let us look at some of the primary concrete activities Mr. Sasakawa has carried out to address these problems associated with leprosy. The first was the holding of a Forum 2000 conference as a venue to teach influential global world leaders about leprosy. The second was the Global Appeal, through which influential people and organizations send a message to eliminate social discrimination (including subsequent activities carried out by those organizations). The third was to establish a scholarship programme, jointly with the globally known spiritual leader the Dalai Lama, for young people living in leprosy colonies. The fourth was to hold a joint symposium at the Vatican, the headquarters of the Roman Catholic Church and its 1.2 billion members around the world. The following examines the impact and social effect of these activities.

(i) Forum 2000—Is leprosy a disease of the past?

At the 5th Forum 2000 conference held in October 2001 in Prague, Mr. Sasakawa addressed leprosy and human rights for the first time as the WHO Special Ambassador and president of the Nippon Foundation at a major international conference. Forum 2000 had been launched jointly by Mr. Sasakawa, the Czech

Republic President Václav Havel, who had battled communism in the fight for freedom, and the author, Auschwitz survivor and Nobel Peace Prize laureate Professor Elie Wiesel. This internationally known forum aims to facilitate understanding and consider how to address a variety of common global issues arising from the wave of globalization. In response to their invitation, the forum has brought together internationally known leaders of various backgrounds from around the world, including Bill Clinton, Henry Kissinger and F. W. de Klerk from the political sphere, the religious leader the Dalai Lama, heads of foundations and NGOs, academics, philosophers, journalists and dissidents. Forum 2000 conferences have been held annually at Prague Castle since 1997.[4]

The main theme of the 2001 Forum 2000 conference was "Human Rights—Search for Global Responsibility". Mr. Sasakawa used this opportunity to plan a special session titled "Human Rights to Health" and gave a speech on "Leprosy and Human Rights", the first time this issue was addressed on an international stage.

Mr. Sasakawa believed that society in general considered leprosy to be a disease of the past, and that it was being forgotten. Nevertheless, leprosy still exists today, primarily in developing countries, and despite the fact that it is curable, many people affected by leprosy do not receive treatment because they fear discrimination, and then develop physical disabilities. Leprosy is a disease for which early detection and early treatment are important. It is important to spread a correct message. More than anything, people have lived with leprosy since biblical times, and it is a negative legacy of humanity.

In his address, Mr. Sasakawa noted that leprosy has been treated with all of the fear that dwells deep within the hearts of people; the fear towards that which is different. "What is startling," he said, "is that we find this strong sense of exclusion around the world, regardless of country, religion, or culture."[5] He went on to say that we cannot allow this disease to continue to be thought of as special. People must use this huge negative legacy of humanity as an example from which to learn. He called on people not to treat leprosy as a special problem, but rather as a universal human rights issue.

Since then, this has been a common theme throughout Mr. Sasakawa's various activities in his work to teach people about leprosy. The problems of the disease and discrimination have many aspects in common with today's coronavirus (COVID-19) pandemic.

Mr. Sasakawa's session was not limited to leprosy. He also asked Waris Dirie, the Somalian supermodel and activist in the fight against female genital mutilation, and Noerine Kaleeba, a Ugandan activist in opposing discrimination against persons with HIV/AIDS, to join him, to show that similar to other modern diseases, leprosy is a universal problem.

The session was attended by Nobel Peace Prize laureate and future president of East Timor José Ramos-Horta, who was made aware of the problem of leprosy in East Timor by Mr. Sasakawa's speech. Following the speech, he approached Mr. Sasakawa and promised to do all he could to eradicate leprosy upon his return. The effect of Mr. Sasakawa's speech was immediately visible. In fact, East Timor achieved the long-sought goal of eliminating leprosy as a public health problem in 2010.

Mr. Sasakawa placed great hope in the ability of the people who attended Forum 2000 to spread this message. He asked them to use their own local media to discuss leprosy whenever they had the opportunity. The personal connections he cultivated at these conferences also proved helpful later with activities like the Global Appeal. Messages communicated via Forum 2000's own media also led to results. One example is the Shared Concern Initiative (SCI), a group of interested Forum 2000 participants who work together to raise the issue of leprosy and human rights around the world.

Over the nine years from 2005 to 2013, many of the issues SCI dealt with were regional conflicts and political oppression in places like Myanmar, Russia, Ukraine and Venezuela, but there were two nonpolitical issues among them: "Solidarity With Japan", concerning the victims of the March 2011 earthquake and tsunami that devasted northeastern Japan, and in the same year, "Human Rights and Leprosy".

The statement on "Human Rights and Leprosy" was issued by H.R.H. Prince El Hassan bin Talal (Chairman, West Africa North Asia Forum, Jordan), Mr. André Glucksmann (philosopher), Professor Vartan Gregorian (President, Carnegie Corporation of

New York), Mr. Frederik Willem de Klerk (former President, Republic of South Africa, Nobel Peace Prize laureate), Mr. Václav Havel (former President, Czech Republic), Mr. Michael Novak (philosopher), Mr. Yohei Sasakawa, Prince Karel Schwarzenberg (former Minister of Foreign Affairs, Czech Republic), the Right Rev. Desmond Tutu (Nobel Peace Prize laureate) and Professor Grigory Yavlinsky (economist, Russia).[6] There is no way to measure the direct effect of this statement, but we can gauge its importance by looking at these names. Messages from influential leaders carry significant weight, and have a major effect on society. Mr. Sasakawa has used the personal connections he cultivated through Forum 2000 in his other activities, and continues to do so today.

(ii) Submission to the International Herald Tribune

In its 18–19 September 2004 weekend edition, the *International Herald Tribune* (published by the New York Times) printed an article by Mr. Sasakawa titled "Conquering an ancient scourge: Leprosy is not a stigma anymore". Following the Forum 2000 conference, Mr. Sasakawa continued to engage with the United Nations Commission on Human Rights and the Sub-Commission on the Promotion and Protection of Human Rights to eliminate discrimination, and the printing of his op-ed contribution by a major Euro-American news outlet was a major achievement. It was rare for the IHT to accept a submission from a Japanese person with whom it had no connection (Appendix 1). It goes without saying that Mr. Sasakawa received many messages of endorsement and encouragement from people who read the article in Japan and around the world. This certainly had a major impact as well as ripple effects and reinforced Mr. Sasakawa's belief in the use of media to disseminate a correct message.

After this, he put great effort into reaching a wider general audience through submissions to overseas media, press releases for various events, projects and conferences, and press conferences and media seminars. From March to December in 2017, Mr. Sasakawa contributed a series of twenty articles in English about the battle against leprosy to the online news site the

Huffington Post (HuffPost), as part of its Project Zero series of articles to raise awareness around neglected tropical diseases and efforts to fight them. The titles of the articles are as follows:[7]

1. Jose Was Sent Away, Banished to an Institution (21 March 2017)
2. Father Damien Went to Hawaii to Care for Leprosy Patients and Became a Saint (28 March 2017)
3. What Did Che Guevara and John F. Kennedy Have in Common? (31 March 2017)
4. It's Mildly Infectious and Treatable—Yet Patients Still Face Discrimination (7 April 2017)
5. In 1985, Leprosy Was Still a Serious Public Health Problem in 122 Countries (21 April 2017)
6. Song and Dance for Leprosy Education (30 May 2017)
7. Motorcycle Heading Toward a Leprosy-Free World (20 June 2017)
8. False Stories of Leprosy Are Passed Down and Still Circulate (27 June 2017)
9. Legal Systems Have Reinforced Discrimination against Leprosy (19 July 2017)
10. Leprosy and Human Rights (13 August 2017)
11. Religion's Role in Discrimination against Leprosy (19 September 2017)
12. Leprosy as a Metaphor and the Pope's Slip of the Tongue (22 September 2017)
13. Power to People Affected by Leprosy (2 October 2017)
14. Three Million Leprosy Patients Are Still Waiting to Be Discovered (9 October 2017)
15. Social Rehabilitation and the Future of Children in Leprosy Colonies (17 October 12017)
16. Brazil and Its Efforts to Eliminate Leprosy (30 October 2017)
17. Discrimination Even in a Small Village of 23 Pygmies (9 November 2017)
18. The History of Leprosy Hidden on Beautiful Islands (21 November 2017)
19. The Heritage of Leprosy in Japan (20 December 2017)
20. The Last Mile to a Leprosy-Free World (26 December 2017)

2. Establishment of and strategy behind the Global Appeal

The first Global Appeal was launched in 2006 as an initiative to send an international message.[8] Various events are held each year on the last Sunday in January, which is designated as World Leprosy Day. The appeal is issued to a global audience on or near this day as a call to eliminate stigma and prejudice against persons affected by leprosy and their families, and is issued by a group of people or an organization with international influence and reach.

When Mr. Sasakawa launched this initiative, he asked Forum 2000 participants, and in particular Nobel Peace Prize laureates, to participate as a way of adding force to the first Global Appeal. These were the right people to choose, given that they are among the first to come to mind in response to the questions, "Who are the most trusted people in the world, who are interested in humanitarian issues, and who through their own activities are globally recognized leaders?" A message from this group of people would have a major impact that would resonate all around the world. This was an excellent idea, and as a group of leaders who already supported these objectives, Forum 2000 was an ideal venue through which Mr. Sasakawa could ask his old acquaintances in person or by letter to participate.

Mr. Sasakawa explained his intention as follows:

> I was painfully aware that the effect of my own activities to bring global attention to this issue and to eliminate misunderstanding, prejudice and discrimination was limited. I thought I needed a stronger voice to have a greater effect. I therefore asked for help from influential friends I have come to know through my many years of Foundation activities, who share my values and with whom I have worked together in the past. Fortunately, I was able to enlist their assistance.[9]

The first Global Appeal was signed in person at the Forum 2000 Conference in 2005 by former President of the Club of Rome Prince El Hassan bin Talal of Jordan and former President of the Czech Republic Václav Havel. Separately, it was endorsed by Nobel Peace Prize laureates the Dalai Lama, former President of

Ireland Mary Robinson, Professor Elie Wiesel, Archbishop Desmond Tutu, and Mr. Sasakawa's partner in agricultural development in Africa, former US President Jimmy Carter, along with world leaders Brazilian President Luiz Inácio Lula da Silva, former Costa Rican President Oscar Arias, Nigerian President Olusegun Obasanjo and former Indian President R. Venkataraman. Mr. Sasakawa's initial connection with most of these people was through Forum 2000, which later continued to provide other important connections as well.[10]

Having decided on the signatories for the Global Appeal, the next important issues were the location from which to issue the appeal and what message to send to the world. It was important for the message to reach both local communities and the global community. This made it necessary to motivate people to spread the message, and the planning of events around the issuing of the message was an important part of this. The endorsing individuals and organizations were also important for their ability to spread the message, but the ability of the media to do so was even more significant.

The first Global Appeal in 2006 was issued from India, the country with the world's largest number of persons affected by leprosy. The ceremony was held on 29 January, World Leprosy Day, and participants included former Chief Justice of India Y.V. Chandrachud, Chuo University Professor and UN Sub-Commission on the Promotion and Protection of Human Rights member Mr. Yozo Yokota, and founding president of the International Leprosy Union Dr. S.D. Gokhale. Panel discussions were also held featuring persons affected by leprosy from Asian countries including India, Nepal and the Philippines.

In its 29 January issue, *The Times of India* printed a full-page colour version of the Global Appeal statement. The following day, on 30 January, the Indian government announced that it had achieved leprosy elimination at the national level. With fortuitous timing, two major pieces of news about leprosy were reported throughout India on consecutive days.

After the ceremony in Delhi, a group of the participants went to Kolkata and had another appeal issuance ceremony and panel discussion with persons affected by leprosy, in hopes that this would generate further media coverage. Unfortunately, the Kolkata event was only picked up by several domestic print media and did not get international exposure. Although the signatories were famous people, they did not attend the ceremony in person, and the event was planned almost entirely by the Nippon Foundation with assistance from local individuals, instead of being hosted by an influential local partner organization; so it must be said that the event did not have the power to mobilize the media. Nevertheless, the list of signatories including Nobel Peace Prize laureates for the first Global Appeal gave authority to the Global Appeal itself, and helped to attract participants for future Global Appeals. That fact can also be seen as a major achievement of Forum 2000. It was unfortunate that at the time the individual signatories were scattered across the globe and could not gather together under one roof. Today, an online discussion would be possible.

3. Global Appeal achievements

The effect of the Global Appeal has been wider than anticipated. One way this can be seen is by the various recognitions received by Mr. Sasakawa.

International Gandhi Award

In March 2006, soon after the first Global Appeal, the Gandhi Memorial Leprosy Foundation informed Mr. Sasakawa that he had been selected as the recipient of the 2006 International Gandhi Award. The award ceremony was held on 12 April 2007 in Wardha in the Indian state of Maharashtra, where Mahatma Gandhi's ashram was located and where the Gandhi Memorial Leprosy Foundation is headquartered. The ceremony was attended by Indian Vice President Bhairon Singh Shekhawat, who presented the award to Mr. Sasakawa. Mr. Shekhawat was also a guest of honour at the National Conference on the Integration and Empowerment of Persons Affected by Leprosy, which had been led by Mr. Sasakawa in New Delhi in December 2005. The main reasons given for Mr. Sasakawa's selection were the results of his various activities since the 1980s towards leprosy elimination, and the success of the Global Appeal held in January 2006.[11] Mr. Sasakawa also received the Millennium Gandhi Award from the International Leprosy Union, one of India's major organizations addressing leprosy-related issues, in 2001. This award is presented only once every millennium.

Mr. Sasakawa has himself cited Gandhi as a role model in his ongoing work to eliminate leprosy and provide relief to persons affected by leprosy and their families. In his remarks at the award ceremony for the International Gandhi Award in 2007, Mr. Shekhawat quoted Mahatma Gandhi, and these words became a motto for Mr. Sasakawa in his work. Gandhi's words were, "Leprosy work is not merely medical relief; it is transforming frustration of life into joy of dedication, personal ambition into selfless service",[12] and his reply when called to open a leprosy hospital in Dattapur: "Opening a hospital is an ordinary thing. You call someone to do it. I will come to close it."[13] Mr. Sasakawa's work in India has sometimes been referred to as a "second coming of Gandhi".[14] We can imagine that Gandhi's thoughts and actions have had a significant effect on Mr. Sasakawa. This also led to Mr. Sasakawa receiving the 2018 Gandhi Peace Prize from the Indian government in 2019.[15]

(i) Subsequent Global Appeals

Despite the limited impact of the first ceremony in India, the event served as a breakthrough for the Global Appeal becoming a regular annual event. There have been seventeen Global Appeals since then, held in major cities around the world on or around the last Sunday in January, World Leprosy Day. Participating individuals and organizations and the location of each ceremony are listed below. Each time, the endorsing organization or individuals have been strategically chosen after careful deliberation for their global activities among the non-leprosy community and influence in local communities, so that the message will spread to all corners of society. These organizations are not asked to contribute funds, but rather to play a major role in voicing their support and showing their commitment to addressing issues related to leprosy and discrimination, and their decision to participate is made by their board of directors or similar decision-making body.

2007	Representatives of people affected by leprosy around the world	Manila
2008	International human rights organizations	London
2009	World religious leaders (Representing Christianity, Judaism, Islam, Buddhism, etc.)	London
2010	World business leaders	Mumbai
2011	World's leading universities	Beijing
2012	Members of the World Medical Association	São Paulo
2013	Members of the International Bar Association	London
2014	National human rights organizations	Jakarta
2015	International Council of Nurses	Tokyo
2016	Junior Chamber International	Tokyo
2017	Inter-Parliamentary Union	New Delhi
2018	Disabled Peoples' International	New Delhi
2019	International Chamber of Commerce	New Delhi
2020	International Paralympic Committee	Tokyo
2021	International Trade Union Confederation	Online
2022	Philanthropic foundations	Online
2023	Individuals and organizations attending the International Symposium on Hansen's Disease—"Leave No One Behind"	Vatican

The events featured individual participants in 2006 and 2007: in 2006, global world leaders, including Nobel Peace Prize laureates; and in 2007, persons affected by leprosy from around the world, who do not usually have an opportunity to appear at public events. Over the following years, a theme such as human rights, religion, business, higher education, medicine, law, nursing, sport for persons with disabilities or labour was selected, and the event was held in coordination with associations of parliamentarians, persons with disabilities, business leaders and others. From 2012, with the World Medical Association in particular, partnering together with international specialist organizations with branches around the world has broadened the scope of Global Appeal activities and facilitated the messages' dissemination.

In addition, to the greatest extent possible, the participating international organizations have been asked to cooperate in holding specific activities in their area of specialization, and this has produced some results. The following are examples: the International Bar Association, the International Council of Nurses, the Inter-Parliamentary Union and Disabled Peoples' International.

(ii) Global Appeal with members of the International Bar Association (Global Appeal 2013)

The approach to the International Bar Association (IBA) began in April 2012 with a visit to a person engaged in research on human rights, and the organization's management board made an official decision to cooperate in June. Mr. Akira Kawamura from Japan was the association's president at the time. Preparations proceeded on track with full cooperation from the association's executives and staff. Using his position as president, Mr. Kawamura contacted bar associations and law societies around the world to ask for their endorsement. As a result, forty-six organizations from forty countries signed the Global Appeal.[16]

In her keynote address representing the IBA at the Global Appeal launch ceremony held on 24 January 2013 at the Law Society building in London, Baroness Helena Kennedy (Co-Chair of the International Bar Association's Human Rights Institute) said that the IBA would do two things:

One—to spread awareness among the world's legal profession, across all jurisdictions, about the discrimination on grounds of leprosy that persists AND of the discriminatory laws that reinforce such discrimination.

Two—to bolster the international legal profession to work towards the repeal of such legislation in their respective countries.[17]

IBA Rule of Law Award

The IBA's determination to eliminate discriminatory laws related to leprosy was further strengthened on 23 October 2014, at the association's Annual Conference in Tokyo. This global meeting brought together roughly 6,000 legal professionals from around the world, and at the conference, Mr. Sasakawa was presented with the IBA Rule of Law Award. This award has been presented to eleven individuals since 2004 in recognition of their significant contribution to international justice, human rights and the rule of law. Almost all of the other recipients are judges or other legal professionals. The recipient before Mr. Sasakawa was the then President of the International Criminal Court Judge Sang-Hyun Song in 2012. Mr. Sasakawa was the first Japanese person to win this award.

Presenting the award, IBA President Michael Reynolds recounted Mr. Sasakawa's achievements to the legal professionals gathered from around the world, and declared that the Global Appeal had been a starting point and that the Nippon Foundation and the IBA would work together as partner organizations. In addition, IBA Executive Director Mark Ellis praised Mr. Sasakawa for having worked with the UN's Human Rights Council to mark the 60th anniversary of the proclamation of the Universal Declaration of Human Rights in 2008, by passing a resolution calling for the elimination of discrimination against persons affected by leprosy and their families.[18]

With the Global Appeal as a starting point, Mr. Sasakawa's activities were recognized by the world's legal community through the IBA, creating a common determination to eliminate leprosy-related discrimination and to repeal discriminatory laws.

Repeal of discriminatory laws

Following this, the IBA compiled a detailed list of discriminatory laws, based on information from various leprosy-related organizations, and sent a questionnaire to all of its member national associations asking whether these types of laws existed. The replies from the national bar associations were not very forward looking, stating that those types of laws did not exist or that they did not have the resources to investigate the issue. Nevertheless, the IBA has continued to support the work of the UN Special Rapporteur on the elimination of discrimination against persons affected by leprosy and their family members, and when problems with discriminatory laws have been identified, has brought them to the attention of that country's bar association. Various organizations have also followed through on the IBA's identification of problems with discriminatory laws. In 2015, India's Law Commission presented a report on discriminatory laws to the Indian government (Report No. 256), and the UN Human Rights Council's Advisory Committee has sent out questionnaires on discriminatory laws and analyzed the replies.

Based on that information, the International Federation of Anti-Leprosy Associations (ILEP) has compiled a database of discriminatory laws that still exist throughout the world. According to ILEP's Chief Executive Officer Geoff Warne, ILEP began gathering information on discriminatory laws in 2016, and as of August 2021 had recorded 130 discriminatory laws, which break down as 77 that deal with segregation or separation, 25 related to employment, 10 on immigration, 7 on marriage or divorce, 6 on voting and 5 on public transportation, with 100 of these discriminatory laws being found in India.[19]

In September 2021, Ms. Alice Cruz, who has served as UN Special Rapporteur on the elimination of discrimination against persons affected by leprosy and their family members since 2017, issued a report to the 76th session of the UN General Assembly titled "An unfinished business: Discrimination in law against persons affected by leprosy and their family members" to promote action by member countries.[20] This major movement can be said to have begun with the IBA's involvement with the Global Appeal.

(iii) Global Appeal with the International Council of Nurses (Global Appeal 2015)

Global Appeal 2015 was issued with the International Council of Nurses (ICN). The ceremony was held in Tokyo on 27 January, with then Japanese Prime Minister Shinzo Abe attending. The following day, the persons affected by leprosy from around the world who had participated in the ceremony were invited to tea with the Imperial Couple, and were honoured by having an audience with Emperor Akihito and Empress Michiko. This received extensive media coverage in Japan.

There are roughly 650,000 nurses in Japan and 16 million around the world. As nurses are the people closest to patients, the ICN was asked to participate to give nurses a better understanding of leprosy and have them help to eliminate discrimination and prejudice in their workplaces. With members in more than 130 countries around the world, the endorsement of the ICN gave great significance to the 10th Global Appeal.

As side events to the ceremony, panel discussions were held on three themes: "Leprosy, Medical Care, and Nursing—Inclusive Dignified Care", "Leprosy—A History that Must Not Be Forgotten" and "Leprosy Today and Tomorrow—How Should Society Respond?" The first panel discussion was on the role and contribution of nurses in caring for persons affected by leprosy, from the perspective of nurses. The second was intended to remember the negative legacy of leprosy, including quarantine policies, social ostracization and family separation, and to preserve those memories. The third aimed to consider what people, including persons affected by leprosy, can do about leprosy-related problems, and to explore new possibilities. This was a valuable opportunity to tell the world about the difficult history persons affected by leprosy in Japan have faced.[21]

Receipt of the ICN's Health and Human Rights Award

As a result of the partnership with the ICN for the Global Appeal, Mr. Sasakawa was presented with the ICN's Health and Human

Rights Award on 17 May 2017 at the ICN Congress held in Barcelona, Spain.[22] This award was established in 2000, and is the only award given by the ICN to a person who is not a nurse. The three recipients prior to Mr. Sasakawa were former United Nations High Commissioner for Refugees Sadako Ogata; United Nations Special Envoy for HIV/AIDS in Africa Stephen Lewis; and former United Nations High Commissioner for Human Rights Mary Robinson. Dr. Frances Hughes, who was the ICN's CEO at the time, noted:

> While leprosy is a curable disease, it continues to face many misconceptions, misunderstandings and stigma. As nurses, we understand the importance of equitable access to health services and of educating the public about the disease. The stigma and discrimination felt by individuals can be major barriers to utilizing health services for prevention, diagnosis and treatment. In addition, stigma and discrimination marginalizes those with the disease and affects their ability to fulfill necessary, culturally expected and economically productive roles in society.[23]

Partnering with the IBA and the ICN, two highly influential, international specialist organizations with huge personal and organizational networks, Mr. Sasakawa has continued to disseminate to the world a correct message regarding leprosy, and the fact that the receipt of these awards has sparked media interest can be seen as having a major, if intangible, ripple effect. The issue now is to ensure that this effect is not temporary, but continues.

(iv) Global Appeal in cooperation with the Inter-Parliamentary Union (Global Appeal 2017)

Let us look at the achievements of another Global Appeal—that launched with the endorsement of the Inter-Parliamentary Union (IPU). The IPU has a long history, having been established in Paris in 1889 by members of parliament from France and Britain with the aim of achieving peace and promoting international arbitration. Initially a group of individual MPs, it later grew into an organization of legislative bodies of sovereign nations. Today the IPU is headquartered in Geneva, with 170 member nations.

· At the time of Global Appeal 2017, the IPU's president was Mr. Saber Chowdhury from Bangladesh. The aim of this Appeal was to disseminate correct information about leprosy to legislators around the world through the IPU, to reinforce medical care and social welfare in general for persons affected by leprosy and their families, and to call for the swift repeal of any discriminatory laws still in existence. The ceremony, held in New Delhi, featured a video message from Indian Prime Minister Narendra Modi and was attended by representatives of legislative bodies of Asian countries where leprosy had yet to be eliminated.

In his opening remarks, Mr. Chowdhury, based on his experience of working to repeal discriminatory laws that had been in place in Bangladesh for 100 years, emphasized:

> It is legislators who make discriminatory leprosy-related laws, legislators who repeal them, and legislators who allocate budgets for leprosy-related measures. The role of legislators is to create not only a world without leprosy but also a world without discrimination, by speaking out in their legislatures and in their constituencies, formulating policies, and mobilizing people. That is the spirit of the IPU.[24]

As an effective way to assist the role of legislators, the IPU and the Nippon Foundation jointly published a "Handbook for Parliamentarians". The handbook began with an explanation of what leprosy is, and then went on to outline the status of leprosy and discrimination today, the existence of discriminatory laws, UN resolutions and the existence of Principles and Guidelines, and examples of good practices for the reintegration of persons affected by leprosy into society, with a particular focus on the role to be played by legislators. This tool to promote awareness is a tangible result from the history of the Global Appeal.[25]

(v) Common front with Disabled Peoples' International (Global Appeal 2018)

Another Global Appeal partner was Disabled Peoples' International (DPI). The physical disabilities that can be seen on the hands, feet and faces of persons who receive a late diagnosis of leprosy is a major issue. Of people diagnosed with leprosy, 5.7% receive the diagnosis late and develop a Grade-2 disability, while the figure for children is even higher at 6.8% (both as of 2020).

Nevertheless, persons affected by leprosy who develop disabilities are not included in the disability community, and for a long time, the UN Convention on the Rights of Persons with Disabilities (CRPD), which defines the rights of persons with disabilities, did not extend its benefits to persons affected by leprosy. Given this situation, Mr. Sasakawa formed a partnership with DPI, the world's largest international organization advocating for the rights of persons with disabilities, and work began to include persons affected by leprosy who had developed disabilities in DPI's activities.

As a joint activity, a questionnaire was sent to disability-related organizations in 150 countries around the world in 2014. Those replies showed that of the 15 million people who had received treatment for leprosy over the preceding twenty years, 3 million had developed disabilities as a result of the disease. Of the 85 countries from which replies were received, 73 countries had persons with disabilities as a result of leprosy, but they were members of DPI organizations in only roughly 20% of those countries.[26] Based on this survey, DPI decided to include persons affected by leprosy in its activities.

At the Conference of States Parties to the CRPD held at the UN headquarters in June 2015, DPI and the Nippon Foundation jointly held a panel discussion titled "Voices of People Affected by Leprosy" as a side event, featuring Mr. Sasakawa as well as persons affected by leprosy from India and the United States and representatives of DPI. Through this cooperation, Global Appeal 2018 was issued from India with the endorsement of DPI. This led to a close relationship between the leprosy community and the disability community. Sharing issues and mutual cooperation became major themes. Up until then, the leprosy community had put forth its uniqueness and sought exclusive recognition and support, and was reluctant to cooperate with other partner organizations because of the significant issue of discrimination, so this cooperation with DPI represented a major breakthrough.

These are five examples of the Global Appeal's partnership with international organizations, but cooperation with other partner organizations can also be seen to have made significant achievements. At the very least, the member organizations of those partner organizations and the individual members of those member organizations received a common message about the elimination of leprosy-related discrimination. The problem has been the follow-up: unfortunately, with the exception of the IBA, ICN, IPU, DPI, and Junior Chamber International (JCI), joint activities have not continued beyond the year in which the respective Global Appeal was held. Activities were only carried out during the year of the Global Appeal, and had a strong sense of being transitory. The impact of the message cannot be measured, but it is unfortunate that continuity has not been seen in subsequent concrete activities. We can expect this issue to be addressed through more effective cooperation with partner organizations in the future.

4. Cooperation with the religious world

(i) Interaction with the 14th Dalai Lama and the scholarship programme

The 14th Dalai Lama has issued numerous statements calling for the elimination of leprosy and discrimination in response to requests from Mr. Sasakawa. Forum 2000 played a major role in these exchanges. The two men first met at a Forum 2000 conference in October 2000, where they were introduced through their mutual friend former President Václav Havel. They have met numerous times since then, and the Dalai Lama participated in Global Appeal 2006 by submitting the message: "I hereby acknowledge and support the Global Appeal on Leprosy and Discrimination which will be announced on January 30, 2006, to the world, in order to enhance elimination of the unjustifiable discrimination toward leprosy affected people" (14 December 2005). He also participated in Global Appeal 2009 by submitting the following message on 18 January:

> People affected by leprosy must be given physical relief, but providing human warmth and a sense of value are equally important.

> I pray this Global Appeal will encourage a greater awareness that real care of the sick does not begin with drugs and medication, but with the simple gift of affection and love.[27]

In August 2012, Mr. Sasakawa had the opportunity to visit the Dalai Lama personally at Dharamshala, India, where the Tibetan government-in-exile is located. During that meeting, he told Mr. Sasakawa of a visit he had made to an ashram set up by Baba Amte for persons affected by leprosy, and noted that what impressed him most was how the people there who were affected by leprosy or had disabilities lived with self-respect. He also mentioned a visit he had made to Orissa (now Odisha) state roughly twenty years earlier with his late brother. At the time, there were roughly 500,000 persons affected by leprosy living in Orissa. He and his brother discussed what they could do, but because 500,000 people was such a large number, they were unable to do anything. He said that it was wonderful that the number had come down, especially in India. Infectious diseases like tuberculosis were treated with quarantine. With leprosy, however, even after a person was cured, they continued to face discrimination and ostracism. He noted that this was not good, and that social habits must change. Religious leaders must call on society to show compassion. Isolation was totally wrong. Society must embrace these people, rather than rejecting them.[28]

Baba Amte was born into an affluent family and embarked on a career in law. One day, he saw a person affected by leprosy lying by the side of a road, but did not stop to help that person. He later regretted this, and the incident led him to spend the rest of his life supporting persons affected by leprosy. He created a community called Anandvan (Forest of Happiness) in Warora in the state of Maharashtra, where persons affected by leprosy and their families could live independently, and he supported those people. He and the Dalai Lama became friends, and this led the Dalai Lama to develop a strong interest in reintegrating persons affected by leprosy and their families into society.[29]

At their meeting in Dharamshala, the Dalai Lama made a proposal to Mr. Sasakawa. He suggested that the two of them, together with his friend and former Indian President Abdul Kalam, visit one of India's 800 leprosy colonies. Members of the media would be invited, and this would increase people's awareness of the issue. The visit took place on 20 March 2014 to a colony in Tahirpur, outside Delhi. On that occasion, the Dalai Lama donated 1 million rupees to the colony, and promised to support it for five years. Then, Mr. Sasakawa proposed that they establish a scholarship programme, with additional funds from the Nippon Foundation, to educate promising young second- and third-generation colony residents. The Dalai Lama's visit received extensive media coverage, and the video has been viewed on the Internet more than 7 million times. This sent a major message to people who did not know about leprosy.

To date, this scholarship programme has given 124 young people in leprosy colonies in nine Indian states the opportunity to pursue higher education at colleges or technical schools. Of the twenty-one students selected in the programme's first two years (2015–16), six have become medical practitioners (including two nurses), four have taken jobs in the tourism industry (one at an airline company and three at hotels), one at an electrical and technology company, one at a marketing company, one at a mining venture, one at an online education provider, one in the manufacturing industry, one in the hospitality industry (at a bakery), four as teachers (including in non-formal education) and one with a local government. Two of the first-year students earn at least 50,000 rupees/month and six earn at least 20,000 rupees/month.

Receiving an education and gaining specialist knowledge has opened the door to employment for young people who would otherwise be denied employment opportunities simply because they were born in leprosy colonies. Scholarship programmes to support the education of young people from these colonies, and those set up by globally influential religious leaders like the Dalai Lama in particular, have cast a significant light on these young people, and have important social significance as well. Born into the impoverished environment of the colony, these young boys and girls with family members affected by illness have no opportunities, and some live their entire lives in the colony and are forced to beg for daily necessities. This support for these downtrodden young people gives them the possibility of overcoming prejudice and discrimination and integrating into society. Mr. Sasakawa's years of friendship with the Dalai Lama, and the exchanges of ideas and sharing of problems that have taken place between them, have created significant achievements like this. Using the donation from the Dalai Lama for an ongoing programme in his name, rather than for a one-time activity, has brought the issue of leprosy and the plight of persons affected by leprosy and their families to the attention of society and succeeded in achieving wider and deeper understanding. This scholarship programme has been administered by the Sasakawa-India Leprosy Foundation (S-ILF). The impact and influence of the words and actions of a religious leader who is looked up to around the world cannot be measured. Seeing this tremendous effect, Mr. Sasakawa has maintained his friendship with the Dalai Lama and will continue to do so.

(ii) International symposium with the Vatican

There is another religious leader whose words and deeds receive global attention—Pope Francis. There have been problems with the Pope's words and deeds with regard to leprosy. After Mr. Sasakawa took action by making public criticisms in the media, a cooperative relationship with the Vatican slowly developed. As a result of this, on 9 and 10 June 2016 a symposium titled "Towards Holistic Care for People with Hansen's Disease, Respectful of their Dignity" was held at the Vatican in Rome.

The conference was jointly held by the Vatican and the Nippon Foundation. The Nippon Foundation had already had a relationship with the Pontifical Council for Health Care Workers (the Vatican's equivalent to a Ministry of Health). The Council had received the Sasakawa Health Prize from the WHO in 1990 in recognition of the community work of Catholic nuns, and in 2009 Cardinal Javier Lozano Barragán was one of the global religious leaders who signed the Global Appeal. The president of the Pontifical Council for Health Care Workers also issues a message each year without fail on the last Sunday of January, World Leprosy Day, calling for the relief of persons affected by leprosy. Despite this knowledge and interest in leprosy, in 2013 Pope Francis issued contradictory messages, using the term "leprosy" as a derogatory metaphor, such as "Careerism is a leprosy, a leprosy", "The court is the leprosy of the papacy" and "Paedophilia is a leprosy infecting the Catholic Church." Mr. Sasakawa became concerned that this would promote an incorrect understanding of leprosy among the general public, and wrote several letters to the Pope asking him to refrain from using the term in this way.[30] These petitions from Mr. Sasakawa to Pope Francis received wide media coverage in Japan and overseas. Nevertheless, the reply from the Vatican only stated that the letters had been received, and they did not appear to have reached the Pope himself.

In June 2015, the Nippon Foundation was informed that a well-known bishop who was close to MORHAN, an organization of persons affected by leprosy in Brazil, had arranged for a group to attend the regular Wednesday Mass for the general public at the Vatican, which is attended by thousands of people, and that there might be an opportunity to have an audience with the Pope. Mr. Sasakawa decided to provide the travel expenses for several of these MORHAN representatives, and also delegated Mr. Tatsuya Tanami, the Nippon Foundation's Executive Director responsible for leprosy-related activities at the time (and the author of this chapter), to join them. Instead of another letter of protest, he entrusted Mr. Tanami with a letter proposing that the Vatican and the Nippon Foundation hold an international conference.

The Mass was held on 17 June in St. Peter's Square, and after the roughly hour-long service concluded, the Pope descended from the stage and faced the congregation, and individually greeted the persons affected by leprosy from Brazil, who were in the fourth row. Mr Tanami was in the middle of the row, and used this opportunity to explain the Nippon Foundation's fight against leprosy and to ask the Pope not to use discriminatory language, and handed him the letter from Mr. Sasakawa. There was no reply for some time, but early the next year, Mr. Sasakawa received a reply dated 12 January from the president of the Pontifical Council for Health Care Workers, Zygmunt Zimowski, informing Mr. Sasakawa that he had agreed to co-host a two-day meeting in the Vatican City on 9 and 10 June 2016. The year 2016 happened to be when the Jubilee for the Sick and Persons with Disabilities was to be held, and the conference attendees would be able to attend the special Mass to be held by the Pope on 12 June. Mr. Sasakawa immediately sent Mr. Tanami back to the Vatican, where he had his first meeting on 8 February.

There were only four months to prepare, but through the efforts of the Nippon Foundation staff and with the full cooperation of leprosy advocacy groups and organizations of persons affected by leprosy from around the world, the international symposium was held at the Vatican as planned in June. The symposium was titled "Towards Holistic Care for People with Hansen's Disease, Respectful of their Dignity", and was jointly held by the Pontifical Council for Health Care Workers, the Good Samaritan Foundation and the Nippon Foundation. Representatives of persons affected by leprosy and religious leaders from around the world gathered under the same roof for the first time to discuss religion's relationship with leprosy. Roughly 250 people from forty-five countries, comprising persons affected by leprosy, religious leaders, members of the United Nations Human Rights Council Advisory Committee, medical experts and representatives of NGOs, attended. Representatives of the Roman Catholic Church, Judaism, Islam, Hinduism and Buddhism presented religious interpretations of leprosy and examples of relief.

Persons affected by leprosy from Japan, India, Brazil, Ghana, China, South Korea, the Philippines and Colombia also spoke, presenting their life stories and efforts to eliminate discrimination. The second day, 10 June, featured a session with persons affected by leprosy and members of the United Nations Human Rights Council Advisory Committee. They discussed the situation with regard to leprosy-related discrimination in various countries, giving the members of the Advisory Committee a chance to confirm the extent to which the Principles and Guidelines were being implemented, making this an important session, with persons affected by leprosy being able to speak directly with human rights specialists.[31] At the end of the second day, a summary of the discussions and presentations was issued as "Conclusions and Recommendations".[32]

WHY PUBLIC AWARENESS MUST BE PROMOTED

On Sunday, 12 June, a special Mass, the Jubilee for the Sick and Persons with Disabilities, was held by the Pope in St. Peter's Square as a special event for the Jubilee Year of Mercy. Roughly 70,000 persons with disabilities, medical practitioners, people involved in social welfare, Christians and members of the general public attended, and listened intently to Pope Francis's words.

During the Mass, Pope Francis noted: "An international conference for persons affected by leprosy has been held in Rome. I am grateful to the organizers and participants and welcome them, and it is my earnest desire that this will bear fruit in the fight against this disease", and this was met with loud applause. The message from the symposium would be spread through the Church to local communities. It would also be delivered at conferences of religious leaders. A message about the elimination of leprosy-related discrimination from the Vatican, headquarters of the world's roughly 1.2 billion Roman Catholics, should carry significant influence. The conference minutes and the Conclusions and Recommendations were printed in English and Italian in the *Journal of the Pontifical Council for Health Care Workers* (no. 90), and distributed around the world.

The Conclusions and Recommendations to emerge from the conference were significant for their ripple effect. The document clearly spelled out the role of religious leaders towards the elimination of leprosy-related discrimination: it would be distributed to the churches of 1.2 billion Roman Catholics around the world, and would also reach leaders of other religions, so it could be expected to reach a wide audience, and by stating that leprosy should not be used as a discriminatory metaphor can be seen as including an expression of remorse on the part of the Pope. This is a valuable and important guideline for people's actions, on a par with UN resolutions and the Principles and Guidelines, and being conveyed through the words and deeds of religious figures is having a significant effect. In addition, the fact that the Vatican itself has a better understanding and awareness can be seen in its subsequent messages.

That evening, Mr. Sasakawa appeared on the Italian 24-hour television news station TGCOM24's programme "Stanze Vaticana" with the Secretary of the Pontifical Council for Health Care Workers, providing an opportunity to inform many viewers about leprosy-related issues. The programme introduced some excerpts from the "Leprosy in Our Time" video of the Nippon Foundation available on YouTube, which presents Mr. Sasakawa's on-site activities related to leprosy. The programme is watched by many people in Italy, and was a significant opportunity to introduce leprosy, the Nippon Foundation and Mr. Sasakawa to a wide audience.

Six months after the symposium, on 29 January 2017 (World Leprosy Day), the Pope said the following during the general Mass in St. Peter's Square after the Angelus prayer:

> Today we celebrate World Leprosy Day. This disease, although in decline, is still among the most feared, and afflicts the poorest and most marginalized. It is important to fight this disease, but also against the discrimination that it engenders. I encourage all those engaged in assisting and in the social reintegration of people suffering from Hansen's Disease, for whom we assure our prayers.[33]

This message was clearly an extension of the previous year's international symposium and the Conclusions and Recommendations. On the previous day, 28 January, the prefect of the Dicastery for Promoting Integral Human Development, Cardinal Peter Turkson, released a message on behalf of the Vatican for World Leprosy Day. The message was titled, "The eradication of leprosy and the reintegration of people afflicted by hanseniasis: a challenge not yet won", and it referred to the previous year's symposium, noting that "It was further emphasized that given their role, it is important for the leaders of all religions, in their teachings, writings and speeches, to contribute to the elimination of discrimination against people afflicted by Hansen's disease." The message stressed that

> We should all commit ourselves—and at all levels—to ensuring that in all countries policies relating to the family, to work, to schools, to sport, and policies of every other kind, that directly or indirectly discriminate against these people are changed, and that governments develop implementing plans that involve people with this disease.[34]

The following year, on World Leprosy Day 2018, Cardinal Turkson again issued a message on behalf of the Vatican that, based on the Conclusions and Recommendations, called for churches, religious communities, international organizations, governments, large foundations, and non-governmental organizations to join the forces to repeal discriminatory laws.[35] This showed the achievements of the symposium over two consecutive years. Again, on World Leprosy Day 2021, the same Cardinal Turkson issued another message on behalf of the Pope. In this, Pope Francis "offered words of encouragement to missionaries, health workers, and volunteers committed to serving those affected by the disease". He also noted that the COVID-19 pandemic "has confirmed the need to protect the right to health for those who are most fragile", and said he hoped "that the leaders of nations will unite their efforts to treat those suffering from Hansen's disease and for their social inclusion".[36]

In his 2021 message, Cardinal Turkson also introduced the "Beat Leprosy" goal, commenting, "Beating leprosy involves more than a mere medical struggle. It also seeks to eliminate the social stigma that accompanies this difficult illness and ultimately envisions the restoration of the human person in an integral way."[37]

This shows how the Nippon Foundation's cooperation with the Vatican came about in a very interesting way, beginning with Mr. Sasakawa's objection to the Pope's use of discriminatory language. Also, the opening of that path towards cooperation was in large part due to the mediation of a prominent Brazilian clergyman who was close to persons affected by leprosy. I believe the trigger was the fact that the Pope actually heard the plea of the persons affected by leprosy at the Vatican, when the request was made to carry out Mr. Sasakawa's idea of jointly holding an international symposium. The fact that 2016 was the "year of the sick" was also a major reason for the Vatican's acceptance. The timing was fortuitous.

Traditionally, the president of the Vatican's Pontifical Council for Health Care Workers issues a message almost every year on World Leprosy Day, calling for aid to persons affected by leprosy and the eradication of the disease. Clearly, however, the international symposium was the trigger for the Vatican's greater awareness of leprosy, and in particular, the Vatican's clearer response to the problems of social discrimination and human rights has been a major step forward. In addition, the spread of that message to the world's 1.2 billion Roman Catholics has major significance. The Second International Symposium on Leprosy at Vatican with a theme, ""Leave No One Behind," was held from 23-24 January 2023. The event was organized by the French Raoul Follereau Fondation, the Italian Association Amici di Raoul Follereau and Sasakawa Leprosy (Hansen's Disease) Initiative, in collaboration with the Dicastery for Promoting Integral Human Development of Vatican. The symposium marked a follow-up to the International Symposium held in 2016. The symposium also featured a launch ceremony for the "Global Appeal 2023 to End Stigma and Discrimination against Persons Affected by Leprosy," which was endorsed by the organizers and participants of the symposium. After the symposium, on 26 January, Mr. Yohei Sasakawa had an audience with Pope Francis and made a request to the Pope for his support for the elimination of leprosy and the prejudice and dis-crimination associated with the disease.

Conclusion: Development of new public awareness activities and cooperation with new partners

The preceding examples demonstrate the success of public aware-ness activities as important tactical elements of Mr. Sasakawa's fight against leprosy.

First, as noted at the beginning of this chapter, Mr. Sasakawa's awareness of the problem stemmed from a concern about the lack of knowledge and misunderstanding of leprosy among the general pub-lic. Mr. Sasakawa's motto consists of three messages—"leprosy is curable", "treatment is free" and there is therefore no need for fear, and "discrimination cannot be tolerated"—but as simple and clear as this information is, it was not reaching the general public. That lack of knowledge among the general public is the source of the fear and apprehension about leprosy that leads to discrimination. If the cor-rect information can be conveyed, the rate of treatment will rise, cases of physical disabilities will decrease and prejudice will disap-pear. The challenge, then, is how to convey that knowledge.

Mr. Sasakawa believed that the method to do this involved six components: 1) Have political leaders gain a correct understanding, and have government policies reflect that and pass on that information through government public relations; 2) Have persons affected by leprosy who no longer require treatment speak out and shed a light on their situation in their local communities; 3) Make effective use of the media; 4) Have influential individuals and organizations from outside the leprosy community disseminate correct information; 5) Encourage influential individuals and organizations from outside the leprosy community to participate in activities to combat social discrimination; and 6) Have influential religious leaders disseminate correct information.

To achieve these objectives, Mr. Sasakawa skillfully reconfigured the networks and connections that he himself, the Nippon Foundation and related organizations had built up over the years. This was not an easy task. First, as the movement's standard-bearer, Mr. Sasakawa had to garner a high level of empathy and confidence to get people to follow him. His activities around the world as WHO Goodwill Ambassador for Leprosy Elimination, personal involvement with international institutions like Forum 2000, his building of cooperative relationships with religious leaders, and awards from prestigious organizations like the Indian government and the International Bar Association recognizing his activities and achievements, have played an important role in building that confidence.

Personal connections made through Forum 2000 were highly influential in areas including the Global Appeal, joint activities with the Dalai Lama and media dissemination. Without those connections, it would be impossible to have Nobel Peace Prize laureates and other social leaders think and speak out about the disease of leprosy and the problem of discrimination. Forum 2000 was a valuable venue for building integrity for Mr. Sasakawa and the Nippon Foundation, and for gaining the confidence of people like Nobel Peace Prize laureates in order to enlist them to resolve to address social issues. In particular, Mr. Sasakawa's friendship with the late President Havel was based on a strong relationship of mutual trust, and Mr. Havel's support was able to generate widespread approval of Mr. Sasakawa's activities.

The annual themes of Forum 2000, including the negative aspects of globalization, democratization and inequality, and human rights crises, resonate deeply with the issue of leprosy, which has been a cause of suffering since prehistoric times and still exists today, and this created empathy among forum participants. The fact that leprosy and discrimination have taken up a position as one of humanity's issues facing modern society is very significant. This is creating an awareness that leprosy is in fact not a unique, minor disease from the past that can be forgotten like an old movie, but is rather a problem that needs to be addressed as a fundamental example of human society's "infringement of human rights through discrimination based on a disease". Forum 2000 participants have responded sensitively to the fact that leprosy is a problem that represents a universal human practice of discriminating against and ostracizing from society people for reasons that are no fault of their own.

These personal connections led to the Global Appeal. The leaders who endorsed the first Global Appeal were all people who were strongly connected to Forum 2000. Their stature also gave major significance to and confidence in the Global Appeal initiative and helped in engaging future endorsees. Enlisting these internationally renowned intellectual leaders and public speakers has been an important tactic in gaining the understanding and support of society at large towards the resolution of this major issue.

The Dalai Lama has been a staunch ally as a public speaker, religious leader and tireless humanitarian activist. He has delivered compassionate messages bringing attention to society's downtrodden, and is known for his action. The Dalai Lama has been pained by the issue of leprosy for many years through his long friendship with Baba Amte, who set up self-sufficient colonies for persons affected by leprosy. After meeting Mr. Sasakawa at Forum 2000 and learning of his tireless efforts to eradicate leprosy, the Dalai Lama has constantly been supportive of Mr. Sasakawa. The Dalai Lama is well aware that society will respond to his actions, and his suggestion to visit a leprosy colony was made with the awareness that it would have an impact on general society. The media response to the visit was significant and went beyond India, with millions of people around the world seeing the Dalai Lama, via internet media, taking the hands of and embracing persons affected by leprosy. Taking up the proposal that his donation be used to fund a scholarship programme to help young people in the colonies can also be seen as a long-term rather than a temporary achievement. The fact that the programme is named after the Dalai Lama also gives the programme high social recognition. It functions as a source of empowerment for young people.

The joint symposium with the Vatican played a major role in using the influence of religious leaders to educate the general public with correct knowledge. The Roman Catholic Church has taken a position of religious love towards persons affected by leprosy and their families, which has long been recognized through the Vatican's messages on World Leprosy Day. However, this has been a message of divine love towards persons affected by leprosy as people who are weak and sick, and the Church's own actions have focused on assisting the weak. The international symposium held with the Nippon Foundation can be seen as having expanded that stance by entering a new phase of protecting the human rights of persons affected by leprosy and supporting their integration into society. The Conclusions and Recommendations that resulted from the symposium called for an end to the use of discriminatory language that reinforces stigma, in particular the term "leper", and urged that the term "leprosy" not be used in a metaphorical sense, as the Pope had previously done. The Conclusions and Recommendations also shed light on the elimination of discrimination and protection of the dignity and human rights of persons affected by leprosy, which the Church had not previously addressed that much. Since the symposium, the Vatican's messages have taken on a clear change in tone, with a focus on protecting human rights and the problem of discrimination.

The Global Appeal has been successful because it has taken a novel approach, working with partners who are internationally influential and consequential but who had not previously been involved with leprosy, and calling for the world to create a society in which leprosy-related discrimination does not exist and to take necessary action to achieve this. Matters that had previously been handled vertically within the leprosy community are now being addressed taking a horizontal approach, as the Global Appeal has succeeded in having individuals and organizations who are not part of the leprosy community send a message that cuts across society. The individuals and organizations who were strategically chosen as partners have high name recognition and the ability to communicate to society at large, and this has made them effective. The fact that they recognize the importance of the problem of leprosy and have joined a global movement, despite leprosy not being their top priority, is the result of the steady efforts of Mr. Sasakawa and the Nippon Foundation, which had already achieved global credibility. These efforts of influential individuals and organizations can be seen as having had a significant impact on society. Although not all of them have subsequently carried on with this work, a number of concrete follow-up activities continue. This can be expected to build even more momentum going forward.

It is difficult to measure the results of these efforts to promote social awareness. Perceiving a visible difference between today and yesterday is not possible. We would like to think that, at the very least, we are leaving an impression on many people that is contributing to a change in mindset. What is certain, however, is that this multifaceted approach to changing society is gradually correcting people's mistaken conceptions. The fact that many organizations, including the WHO, national governments, the IBA and the ICN, have recognized Mr. Sasakawa's efforts and honoured his work is proof of this. The many arrows that Mr. Sasakawa has fired have certainly hit the invisible target, and the results of his efforts are beginning to be seen.

* * *

Appendix 1: Excerpt from Yohei Sasakawa, "Conquering an Ancient Scourge: Leprosy is Not a Stigma Anymore", International Herald Tribune, 18–19 September 2004.

For millennia, societies around the world have been terrified by leprosy. But this fear has been nothing compared with the life of sheer abjection that those affected by the disease have had to face.

So those of us working toward the elimination of the disease were thrilled when the 56th United Nations Sub Commission on the Promotion and Protection of Human Rights, meeting in

Geneva on Aug. 9, adopted a resolution entitled, "Discrimination against leprosy victims and their families." It seemed that the mountain had finally started to move.

Most people have never even seen a person with leprosy and in most countries the disease is no longer a public health issue. But... discrimination continues, and in heinous forms. ... not just toward those with the disease, but their families as well.

Since the development in the early 1980s of multidrug therapy, which can defeat leprosy within six months to a year, 13 million people have been cured. The number of nations where leprosy is endemic has plummeted from 122 to about six.

The leprosy of today is milder than the flu. If treated quickly, it appears as nothing more than a localized skin rash. ... In fact, most of the world's leprosy patients have been cured permanently. But the disease continues to cause one of the most horrible forms of discrimination known to humanity: lifetime banishment.

... Even those who have been cured are often unable to return to their places in the community... They find it difficult to marry, to get work and to go to school.

In an effort to escape disgrace, families will often cast out members who have contracted the disease... These individuals, disowned utterly, are turned out of their homes, stripped of their names and even denied a place in the family grave.

7

LEPROSY CONTROL IN THE POST-ELIMINATION ERA

Marcos Virmond

Leprosy as a neglected tropical skin disease

Leprosy and other infectious diseases are part of our world biome. Many of these diseases are threatening to human beings and, since the beginning of time, empiric or scientific measures have been proposed by lay people, priests, wise men, doctors and scientists to halt their jeopardizing effects. Some of the classical diseases still affecting humans are ancient; others have disappeared due to the natural declining course of the causative agent. Concerning still others, we have just a faint idea of their existence through the narrative of historians, as in the case of the sweating sickness, a devastating illness that briefly reached epidemic proportions in some countries in Europe in the fifteenth and sixteenth centuries.[1]

It takes time to understand which pathogen is responsible for a given disease, its behaviour, weaknesses and strong points. However, the inquietude of humanity drives us to seek information and knowledge to control, and preferably eliminate, the causative agent, if applicable. In this sense, throughout the history of humanity advances in technical knowledge have strongly modified the health condition of populations, improving their quality of life and life expectancy. New drugs and new vaccines are offered for old and even new, emerging diseases, whose natural history and epidemiology—in the case of the latter—are scarcely known.

Thus, elimination or eradication of human diseases has been a dream of doctors and politicians, while the topic has been the subject of numerous conferences, workshops, symposiums and public health initiatives for more than a century. Indeed, as knowledge advances, public health personnel are encouraged to rethink old strategies and to propose measures to counter the effects of disease on populations, prevent disease, and allow equitable social development. As George Crabbe wrote in his "The Borough"—Letter I (1810) , adapted by Montagu Slater to a libretto for Benjamin Britten's opera Peter Grimes,

> In ceaseless motion comes and goes the tide
> Flowing it fills the channel broad and wide
> Then back to sea with strong majestic sweep
> It rolls in ebb yet terrible and deep.

> Montagu Slater, Peter Grimes, Act III, Scene 2

Elimination of tropical diseases

To eliminate a disease some clear concepts and criteria must be established. Eradication of infectious diseases involves reducing worldwide incidence to zero, thereby avoiding the need for further control measures. In its turn, elimination can be approached in two ways: elimination of transmission or elimination as a public health problem.

The two terms must not be mistaken for one another. The former means reduction to zero of the incidences of infection caused by a specific pathogen in a defined geographical area, with minimal risk of reintroduction, as a result of deliberate efforts, and may require continued actions to prevent re-establishment of transmission. The latter is a term related to both infection and disease. It is defined by achievement of measurable global targets set by the World Health Organization (WHO) in relation to a specific disease. When reached, continued actions are required to maintain the targets and/or to advance the interruption of transmission.[2]

In brief, elimination of infectious diseases involves reducing morbidity to a level at which they are no longer considered a major public health problem. Elimination still requires a basic level of control and surveillance. Differing from eradication, an inaccurate concept such as elimination needs the adoption of a given standard to be achieved. The definitions of elimination as a public health problem, as well as the indicators used to assess their achievement, are specific to each disease and should be carefully established after a consultative process by national health authorities, the scientific community and the WHO. In addition, geographical levels of attainment should be defined, such as elimination at country, regional or global level.

Elimination of an infectious disease involves both biological and non-biological issues. The latter are mainly social and politically related issues; the former are self-explanatory and mostly dependent on a clear concept of what constitutes a case, a standardization of diagnosis in field conditions and a reliable, robust and accessible drug treatment.[3]

Elimination of leprosy as a disease

Leprosy is among the group of neglected tropical diseases targeted by WHO for eradication, elimination of transmission or elimination as a public health problem, at regional or global level, together with Chagas disease, human African trypanosomiasis, dog-mediated human rabies, lymphatic filariasis, onchocerciasis, schistosomiasis, trachoma, visceral leishmaniasis and yaws.[4]

With regard to leprosy, the biological factor supporting WHO's setting of an elimination target included the existence of a new and robust drug regimen to treat leprosy infection, i.e., the multidrug therapy (MDT) regimen. After a long and not fully successful use of dapsone monotherapy, in which patients had to take daily pills for life, the adoption of the MDT regimen has also drastically changed the concept of cure of leprosy. It was time for leprosy to shed its historical image as a frightening, incurable and stigmatizing biblical disease.

An additional reason for the success of MDT can be credited to the development of blister packs, which greatly facilitated distribution and drug taking. The blister presentation was jointly developed by Dr. Yo Yuasa and Dr. Hiroshi Nakajima.[5] The former was Executive and Medical Director of the Sasakawa Health Foundation (then known as the Sasakawa Memorial Health Foundation) and the latter served as the WHO Director-General from 1988 to 1998. A wider implementation of MDT was facilitated by further modification of the technical and managerial aspects of MDT, such as the adoption of a simplified classification of leprosy into multibacillary (MB) type and paucibacillary (PB) type on clinical grounds.

The challenge of eliminating a disease

Depending on the geographical area, the time frame in which the goal of elimination may be attained will vary. So, the concept of elimination must be approached from an open perspective in terms of time and boundaries, although not necessarily in terms of its quantitative goal. Elimination is ultimately a mission that requires engaging with committed health agents on a physical, mental and philosophical level. They need more than just basic knowledge of the disease and drugs to deliver; they need to be given moral support as well.

Leprosy, among other transmissible neglected diseases, is a disease for which fulfilment of an elimination goal requires strong support. The reasons are the lack of an effective vaccine, the strong accompanying stigma and discrimination, and the disease's high prevalence among underserved populations. Aside from the misery of those affected by the disease, these aspects also affect those who work with it, thus creating an endless vicious circle that can render both patients and caregivers extremely vulnerable and in need of special support. In this regard, leprosy is unique.

Consequently, leprosy requires an internationally recognized figure to act as a guiding light providing hope to those adrift in a sea of disorientation. That person should inspire both health workers and patients alike—the former to find and treat patients and the latter to believe in the possibilities a cure and a better quality of life. Such a figure is found in the person of the WHO Goodwill Ambassador for Leprosy Elimination.

What has been achieved so far

At the present stage of the control of leprosy, "elimination" is a feasible achievement and "eradication", in the short run, is not. Even though autochthonous cases of leprosy are scarcely seen in highly developed countries nowadays, most likely the result of social and economic progress, to eradicate the disease on a world-wide basis would require a vaccine with reasonable efficacy. Hence, the WHO strategy has focused on the elimination of the disease as a public health problem and not primarily on its eradication.

Three decades after the 44th World Health Assembly adopted a resolution in 1991 to eliminate leprosy as a public health problem by the year 2000, with elimination defined as a prevalence rate of less than one case per 10,000 population, the results are striking. Global prevalence has dropped from 21.1 cases per 10,000 population in 1985 to 0.24 cases per 10,000 population in 2016. In 2020, this figure dropped to 0.16 cases per 10,000 population, confirming that leprosy has long been eliminated at the global level and that "elimination" has been maintained.

Today, only one country, with the exception of some small island states, has yet to declare it has eliminated leprosy as a public health problem. That country is Brazil, which, along with India and Indonesia is still detecting more than 10,000 new cases a year. These case numbers indicate continued transmission of the disease. However, this should not be seen as a defeat of the strategy: these are large, economically and culturally diverse countries with big populations. The possibility of them not attaining the goal was long ago predicted by the WHO authorities when it analyzed their characteristics and the particularities of their endemicity for leprosy. And these countries are quite aware that the fight goes on and that leprosy should not be forgotten.

For a disease with a long incubation period, with—most of the time—only faint signs and symptoms in its early presentation and with serious stigma and prejudice involved, leprosy control and elimination need continuous efforts, dialogue, patience, expertise, funds, knowledge and commitment both by care providers and stakeholders, and the existence of a Goodwill Ambassador is of utmost relevance. His main duty is to keep the momentum going in the face of any difficulties that show up, as they invariably will following initial good results, in a strategy as ambitious as the elimination of leprosy.

An international leader is required

United Nations Goodwill Ambassadors are distinguished individuals, carefully selected from the fields of art, literature, science or other walks of public life, who have agreed to help focus worldwide attention on the work of the United Nations. In promoting health and well-being, the WHO has the capacity to nominate persons in this role. Backed by the WHO Director-General, these prominent personalities volunteer their time, talent and passion to raise awareness of WHO efforts to improve the lives of billions of people worldwide. Considering the political challenges involved in a huge enterprise such as attaining the elimination of leprosy, the appointment of a Goodwill Ambassador would come to be seen as vital to those efforts. Interestingly, however, Mr. Sasakawa's initial appointment as a leprosy elimination ambassador came ten years after the original World Health Assembly resolution in 1991, and one year after the original deadline of 2000 had passed.

In the run-up to that deadline, it had become clear that a number of countries would need more time, and so the deadline was extended to 2005. To help give the elimination strategy a final push, a Global Alliance for the Elimination of Leprosy (GAEL) was established in 1999. The first meeting of GAEL was held in India in 2001. Among the decisions taken at that meeting was the appointment of Mr. Yohei Sasakawa, then president of the Nippon Foundation, as GAEL's Special Ambassador.

His initial task was to achieve two fundamental aims: to obtain the firm commitment of political leaders of endemic countries and to urge them to grasp this opportunity to heighten the priority given to elimination of leprosy within their governments. In addition, Mr. Sasakawa recognized the importance of enlisting the support of the world's media in order to have them disseminate correct information on leprosy, mainly regarding the curability of the disease and the free availability of treatment, and to send the strong message that discrimination should no longer have a place in today's world.

The appointment of Mr. Sasakawa as GAEL Special Ambassador was a step on the path to the WHO Director-General nominating him, in 2004, as WHO Goodwill Ambassador within the legal framework of the United Nations. It was a crucial step to open a new window of opportunity to expand the commitment of the ex-GAEL Special Ambassador to the cause of leprosy elimination and human rights. Indeed, the new position as a formal WHO Goodwill Ambassador would grant Mr. Sasakawa heightened international recognition and smooth the way for him to meet national leaders and stakeholders and deliver his message of hope and conviction concerning the elimination of leprosy.

Leprosy beyond elimination: who needs an ambassador for "elimination"?

By the time of Mr. Sasakawa's appointment as WHO Goodwill Ambassador, all but a handful of countries had achieved the goal of eliminating leprosy as a public health problem, but that did not mean the job was done. Elimination needed to be maintained and further inroads needed to be made against the disease to move ahead towards a world without leprosy. In that sense, Mr. Sasakawa's appointment can be seem as straddling the "elimination" era and what was to follow.

Leprosy elimination was a matter of reducing prevalence, and this could be achieved by caring for and curing people and then removing them from the epidemiological data. The remaining challenge after elimination was reducing incidence, which in leprosy usually is taken as the rate of detection of new cases. It is closely related to reducing transmission of an infectious disease—a hard task.

Therefore a new scenario has opened up in front of the ambassador, requiring innovative approaches to address the remaining burden of leprosy. That is the challenge and, as it is said in Japan, "In a journey of a hundred miles, the 99th mile is no better that half-way." In brief, the last mile of the fight against leprosy is perhaps the most arduous, and that is the chief reason we still need an international leader to stimulate health workers, convince politicians and give voice to the underserved community of leprosy-affected persons. More than ever, there is a need to continue pushing towards a world without leprosy. That is the task for an ambassador for leprosy elimination, even in the post-elimination era.

Early engagement in the fight against leprosy

It is easy for an international leader with sound private institutional support to be engaged in any philanthropic mission. What is difficult and unusual is to maintain lasting commitment, since commitment to a social cause takes time and money and frequently diverts one's attention from one's main interest.

Some people have the impression that Mr. Yohei Sasakawa is seeking to promote himself through his leprosy work. They will point to photos taken on his tours around the world of him visiting authorities, health units and leprosaria, and say it is easy to have a professional photographer make him look good as he kneels before a leprosy patient and embraces him. However, if one looks attentively at such photos, I am convinced that another reading is possible and, indeed, is the truth—that this gesture is a demonstration of compassion.

To understand such potential controversy, let us remind ourselves that in the eighteenth century two famous philosophers and thinkers, Jean-Jacques Rousseau and Adam Smith, stated that sympathy or pity have political and moral importance. Smith recognized that sympathy is the foundation of political harmony and, if properly cultivated, is the basis of cooperative communities, enabling citizens emotionally to attune themselves to each other. Along the same lines, Rousseau contended that pity should be the primary and most important emotion to be cultivated by citizens. He argued that shared suffering creates bonds of affection, leading to a sense of common humanity. In this context, compassion, asserted Rousseau, was the democratic emotion par excellence. This idea was later encapsulated in the new ethical altruism of the positivist Auguste Comte's aphorism, "*vivre pour autrui*" (live for others). It seems to me that compassion is a leading emotion at work amidst Mr. Sasakawa's involvement in the fight against leprosy.

This involvement is of long standing and remains unchanged. It is also expressed by concrete actions in the form of participation in, encouragement of and financial support for core leprosy activities. The involvement goes back to 1974, when Mr. Ryoichi Sasakawa, founder and first president of the Japan Shipbuilding Industry Foundation (JSIF), deeply concerned about the global leprosy situation, began financially supporting the WHO Global Leprosy Programme (WHO/LEP). On receiving a donation of around US$1 million from the JSIF, the WHO Director-General requested that half the amount be earmarked for the small-pox eradication programme, then an immediate priority, and Mr. Sasakawa assented. This was the initial step towards a long and fruitful relationship with WHO.

Of note was the fact that funds were allocated both for direct support for the Global Leprosy Programme and research activities. Among the latter, notable were the initial international trials of multidrug therapy (MDT) conducted in the Philippines, South Korea and Thailand, in response to the recommendation of the International Workshop on Chemotherapy of Leprosy in Asia, which took place in Manila in 1977 to address the increasing problem of dapsone resistance.

Later, the JSIF changed its name to the Nippon Foundation (TNF), and the total amount donated to WHO had reached almost US$4 million by 1980. Separate from this was the remarkable action taken by TNF to guarantee MDT drugs for free global distribution through the WHO to meet the needs of leprosy-endemic countries from 1995 to 1999. The announcement of this additional US$50 million contribution from TNF to help accelerate the global leprosy elimination campaign was made by Mr. Yohei

Sasakawa in July 1994, on the occasion of the first International Conference on the Elimination of Leprosy as a Public Health Problem, held in Hanoi, Vietnam, under the joint sponsorship of the WHO and TNF/SHF. It is doubtful whether the WHO would have been able to succeed in the huge challenge of eliminating leprosy as a public health problem without the additional funds from TNF for supplying free MDT. Since 2000, that drug security has been provided by Novartis.

At the inauguration of the above-mentioned Global Alliance for the Elimination of Leprosy (GAEL) in Abidjan, Côte d'Ivoire, in 1999, Mr. Sasakawa announced a further contribution of US$24 million over the period up to 2005, bringing the total contribution of TNF to the WHO to nearly US$150 million—testimony to a remarkable collaboration. As a matter of fact, TNF remains the major funder of the WHO Global Leprosy Programme (GLP) to this day.

The Bangkok Declaration

In view of the need to sustain leprosy services for a world free of leprosy, a shift was proposed in the approach to the leprosy elimination strategy. The idea was to move from a campaign-like elimination approach towards the process of sustaining integrated, high-quality leprosy services. The basic principles of leprosy control remained the same, namely early detection of cases and treatment with MDT. Perhaps more importantly, this initiative recognized that special expertise in leprosy and its control needs to be maintained at national and sub-national levels. It was emphasized that the key point in the new approach was to integrate all the essential components of leprosy control activities into the available primary health care system. In line with this, the strategy sought to sustain leprosy control activities wherever leprosy existed, helping to uphold the gains made by the elimination strategy and reduce the disease burden further in the still endemic countries.

However, as Mr. Sasakawa travelled the world, he got the clear impression that health ministries were losing interest in leprosy. Indeed, the data showed a worrying mix of stable new case numbers and pockets of high endemicity. Potentially, the dramatic and convincing results of the elimination strategy and its further enhancement were promoting leaders' complacency and risked undoing the hard work to date. Mr. Sasakawa stressed that leprosy had caused untold damage to human beings and that the world was at a critical juncture in the fight against the disease. There was a need to revise the course of action and call for renewed commitment. These were the reasons for the organizing of an International Leprosy Summit in conjunction with the WHO South-East Asia Regional Office.

The summit was held in Bangkok, Thailand, in July 2013, bringing together health ministers and health ministry officials from seventeen countries that annually report over 1,000 new cases of leprosy. Mr. Sasakawa clearly stated that the fight against leprosy was not over and urged governments to use the summit as an opportunity to reaffirm their strong determination to achieve "a leprosy-free world", a phrase that would feature in the title of the subsequent "Bangkok Declaration" and became a landmark of the summit.[6]

Despite the impact of the leprosy elimination strategy in dramatically reducing the prevalence and the detection of new cases, many technical and operational challenges remain to be addressed in order to realize a leprosy-free world. Among the technical challenges of note are the following: continued occurrence of new cases; the need to sustain and improve quality of care; the need to guarantee early detection of cases; the need to provide good laboratory services; and the need for reliable control of contacts. Of course, these were not new issues, but new strategies were to be designed to overcome such barriers to a leprosy-free world.

After three days of lively discussions, the summit participants recognized the urgent need to focus on the early detection of new cases in pockets of high risk such as urban slums, border regions and ethnic minority areas. In addition, participants agreed on the goal of reducing the number of new cases with Grade-2 (visible) disability to less than one case per million population by 2020, and to create a mechanism in each country to monitor and evaluate the effectiveness of anti-leprosy activities. Other crucial points agreed included access to equitable and quality health care, including rehabilitation and referral systems.

It was an important moment for countries to renew their commitment to reducing the burden of leprosy and, most of all, to recognize the importance of the involvement and participation of individuals and communities of people affected by leprosy, including efforts to reduce stigma and discrimination as a major step to achieving the goal. Of course, the summit also emphasized the need for adequate resources for supporting programme implementation and recognized the continuing need for supporting research in leprosy.

Another important declaration by Mr. Sasakawa came at the end of the meeting. He stressed that elimination of leprosy at the national level was only a milestone; it was not the end of the road. He clearly stated that governments were urged to achieve leprosy elimination within a new framework, that is, at sub-national levels. To attain that, they should not be concerned if the number of cases increased, which is to be expected after strengthening efforts at elimination, due to more cases being diagnosed. This was received with some surprise and relief. Indeed, major endemic countries, such as Brazil and some countries in sub-Saharan Africa, despite their renewed effort to control leprosy, faced difficulties in attaining the goal of elimination even at the national level. Those present applauded the Ambassador's willingness to be flexible, given differences between countries, while not losing sight of the goal of a leprosy-free world.

Later, the Ambassador reiterated his position in his newsletter: "People may be surprised to hear me say that I would like to see an increase in case numbers, but I have my reasons." Indeed, a main criticism of the "elimination" of leprosy was that authorities were focused on lowering the number of cases and neglecting activities that might result in an increase in new case detections, fearing the criticism that might come. Astutely, the Ambassador made clear, again, that "there is nothing to be ashamed of in seeing patient numbers increase".[7]

The summit concluded with the issuing of the "Bangkok Declaration: Towards a Leprosy-free World", signed by all the ministers of health and relevant authorities of participating countries. Against this backdrop, Mr. Sasakawa announced that the Nippon Foundation was committing US$20 million for leprosy control worldwide over a five-year period, including US$3.8 million earmarked for the Bangkok Declaration-related activities through a special fund that became to be known as the Bangkok Declaration Special Fund (BDSF).

The BDSF attracted the attention of many endemic countries. A number of project proposals were submitted and those that were accepted were later conducted under the sponsorship of TNF. The process involved a bottom-up approach with eligible countries submitting a multiyear proposal, which was reviewed by external experts and submitted to the donor. In the Democratic Republic of Congo, a project was started in 2015 that targeted eight provinces with the highest burden of leprosy and difficult-to-access health zones. Its main objective was to increase case detection by 50%, compared to the baseline year 2013. As a preliminary result, in the first year the numbers of new cases detected in the project area exceeded expectations, showing a 73% increase compared to the 2013 baseline. In Nepal, BDSF-supported mini campaigns focused on active case detection covering six districts. As a result, the number of cases detected in the project area doubled.

More exciting was the result of a BDSF project in Brazil, where leprosy is referred to as Hansen's disease. "Innovative approaches to intensify efforts towards a Brazil free of Hansen's disease" targeted nineteen priority municipalities. During the first year of implementation, 5,651 health professionals were trained, among them 834 doctors, involving ninety-five primary health care centres. During in-service training and nineteen subsequent skin campaigns, 207 new cases were diagnosed, of which 20% were children.[8] Indeed, innovation was also a key point addressed by proposals submitted to the BDSF.[9] For South America, innovative approaches to old issues were tackled by approved projects in the area of geo-referencing of index cases and identification of transmission hotspots, and in the implementation of the Explanatory Model Interview Catalogue (EMIC) scale, applied to individuals with stigmatizing conditions in order to measure perceived stigma and self-stigma. The implementation of the EMIC scale is innovative as it can serve as an instrument in gathering the necessary information related to stigma among people affected by leprosy for informed action, as appropriate.

Another relevant project in South America was the introduction of an e-approach to monitoring of reactions to Hansen's disease through the implementation of a Reaction Surveillance System (SISREAÇÃO). This surveillance system appears more innovative, not only for its ability to capture leprosy patients with reactions, but also with its potential to allow for follow-up of patients after discharge from the treatment regimens, based on the knowledge that it is possible for reactions to occur up to one year after the end of treatment. This approach gives patients at risk of developing reactions an extra sense of security, adding additional credibility to the programme.

The same applies to Southeast Asia, where a project on procurement and distribution of mobile handsets to project staff for GPS tracking and mapping of patients, with associated activation of a leprosy helpline, was developed. This proposal may have facilitated easy and prompt communications, enhanced mapping/geo-coordination of cases and resultant follow-up activities in the local leprosy control programme. In Africa, one project proposed the provision of a toll-free telephone helpline to enable patients and members of the public to access information on leprosy on a confidential basis. In fact, a toll-free telephone helpline can prove attractive to the target population, with a resulting improvement in the impact and outcome of the project.

The BDSF follows closely one of the main personal philosophies that guide the actions of Mr. Yohei Sasakawa, namely, "The place where problems occur is also where solutions will be found." Thus, the criteria for funding projects under the BDSF focused on innovation, especially in case detection, surveillance, community involvement, and monitoring and evaluation, mainly in countries with identified shortcomings in leprosy control but with leaders in place, motivated and skilled, to solve them. In this sense, the BDSF was the meeting point between the felt need, local engaged leaders and renewed governmental commitment, all of that encircled by a strong understanding of the need to come together and "walk hand in hand" to achieve a leprosy-free world. As a result, the BDSF was a step forward in the post-elimination effort, that was launched in timely fashion to stimulate governmental leaders whose momentum to go further in tackling leprosy was diminishing.

Travelling in the post-elimination era

Interestingly, the Goodwill Ambassador increased his activities even as the elimination target was progressively attained in countries where leprosy had been a burden. Instead of reducing his commitment to the cause, he continued to travel around the globe offering support to address local needs and encouragement for health personnel to further reduce the leprosy burden. He acted as a diplomatic globetrotter, participating in political and technical meetings, addressing opening ceremonies of scientific societies, but also visiting leprosaria and attentively listening to stories of those affected by leprosy. His presence on the spot can be understood by his personal philosophy: 1) the place where problems are happening is also where solutions will be found; 2) taking action to transform society requires a strong and committed spirit that can withstand hardships; and 3) I must keep going until results are obtained.

Among these principles, the very first one is of most relevance for its close relation to the practical reality of fieldwork, a reality that is seldom recognized by policymakers. Luckily, the Ambassador has taken it as his first philosophical principle. Keeping this concept in mind, it is possible to explore it in relation to its link to incentivizing health workers in the field.

Incentives for health workers can be defined as "an available means applied with the intention to influence the willingness of physicians and nurses to exert and maintain an effort towards attaining organizational goals".[10] Incentives can also be an explicit or implicit financial or non-financial reward for performing a particular act.[11]

Literature discussing incentive schemes in health care stresses that financial incentives alone are not sufficient to motivate health staff. Non-financial incentives, within limits, play an equally crucial role and they are most relevant in countries that have limited funds for the health sector. Literature references confirm that employee engagement has a significant impact on employee performance, and that health workers with high levels of occupational stress tend to have lower work engagement.[12]

This is the case for those professionals working in general health services where providing leprosy care is an additional responsibility among other duties. Of course, fair pay and satisfying benefits also lead to highly engaged employees, but this is seldom the reality in most public health services in endemic countries. However, rewards and recognition are found to be another important determinant for engagement.

That is one facet of the Ambassador's strategy. His frequent physical presence on the spot indicates to local health workers that their commitment to fight leprosy is something appreciable, tangible and relevant, and gives them a strong sense of the crucial contribution they are making towards reducing the leprosy burden.

Thus, a prominent visit by the Ambassador bears witness to their rarely recognized value. And this boost to their morale, on many occasions, is enough to encourage them to refine their services and, ultimately, to strengthen their commitment and engagement to the cause.

Probably because he recognizes this crucial aspect of his role, the Ambassador constantly moves around the globe visiting endemic countries, often returning for follow-up visits. The Ambassador clearly stated his duties at the Global Forum on the elimination of leprosy as a public health problem held in Geneva in 2006.[13] He declared he had three main purposes in making these trips. First, he aims to talk with politicians for whom the elimination of leprosy may not be such a priority and encourage them to give it more attention; second, he makes these trips to solicit the cooperation of the mass media, because they are an important partner in the struggle against leprosy; and third, he travels to encourage people working at the front line. Figure 1 illustrates in numbers this strategy around the six WHO official regions, totalling up to 201 visits in the period. Of note are the number of repeat visits to countries such as India, Indonesia, Nepal and Brazil, where there is still much work to be done to reduce the burden of leprosy. As seen in the same figure, these overseas visits had to be curtailed because of the impact of the COVID-19 pandemic in 2020–21. Instead, the Ambassador sought to fulfill his mission by taking part in webinars to communicate with and encourage national programme officers and persons affected by leprosy.

Of course, the Ambassador's mandate is not restricted to field visits. Another relevant and essential role is his high-level interac-

Figure 1: Number of visits to countries, per WHO region and year (2001–2021)

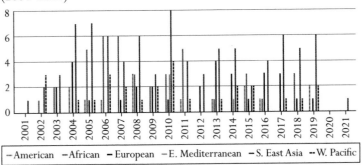

tion with health ministers and, whenever this can be arranged, with presidents and prime ministers. The voice of the Ambassador on behalf of the fight against leprosy and against the discrimination of leprosy-affected persons has been instrumental in stimulating endemic countries to keep leprosy issues on the health agenda.

Sometimes these meetings do not go to plan, as happened in 2015 in Brazil, when Mr. Sasakawa had a difficult exchange with the health minister and his visit was not well received. Mr. Sasakawa subsequently succeeded in repairing relations with the Brazilian government, and during his visit in 2019 he had a fruitful meeting with President Jair Bolsonaro which was live-streamed on Facebook.[14] Fortunately, in most instances, such as his several encounters with the prime minister of India, countries have welcomed the opportunity to meet with Mr. Sasakawa.

These interactions with local country authorities have also been facilitated by National Leprosy Conferences organized by TNF and SHF. Such conferences are an initiative of Mr. Sasakawa, aiming to stimulate the head of state to join the group of participants and thus creating momentum for working on leprosy. It is worth highlighting the National Conference held in Myanmar in 2018 at the Myanmar International Convention Centre-II in Nay Pyi Taw. With the motto "join hands to stop discrimination", the conference focused on human right issues related to leprosy-affected persons. It was a unique opportunity to gather together high-ranking government leaders to secure their commitment to the fight against discrimination and to the care of leprosy patients as a whole. Then State Counsellor Aung San Suu Kyi, the de facto leader of the country, gave the opening address. In 2019, TNF and SHF organized a National Conference in Bangladesh. The conference was inaugurated by Prime Minister Sheikh Hasina, who spoke about the need to treat persons affected by the disease as part of society and not to harbour negative attitudes toward them. It was a direct call for inclusion. More than that, the prime minister urged all relevant authorities, beginning with the Ministry of Health and Welfare, to take concrete steps to achieve "zero leprosy".

The most recent National Conference was scheduled to take place in Brazil in 2020. Although the Brazilian president and the first lady had confirmed their intention to attend, the conference had to be postponed just five days before it was due to begin after Brazil declared a state of emergency to fight the novel coronavirus. The current plan is for the National Conference to be held at the end of 2023 in collaboration with the Lula administration.

The reasons for the success of these encounters with government officials and leaders are not the same as for the field visits. Politicians can be sensitive to some pressure from international authorities, and it is quite possible that by including these meetings on his itinerary, the Ambassador is able to ensure that leprosy receives attention and that countries give some priority to addressing it.

The Ambassador also frequently pays visits to scientific meetings, such as the 12th Brazilian Leprosy Congress held jointly with the ILA (International Leprosy Association) Regional Congress of the Americas in 2011 in Maceió, Brazil. He has also participated in the opening ceremony of the ILA International Leprosy Congress several times, such as the 18th ILA International Leprosy Congress in Brussels in 2013. His presence there was interpreted by participants as a message that the fight against leprosy requires not only clinical expertise and the science that underpins it, but something more. In other words, if the fight against leprosy begins in the questioning mind of the scientist, which offers solutions that must echo in the mind of health policymakers, and which are ultimately applied by health personnel in the field, it requires the advocacy abilities of leaders such as the Goodwill Ambassador to make these relevant and appealing, so as to secure the political commitment of decision makers.

In brief, the Ambassador has travelled to almost 100 countries to learn about problems and solutions at first hand. He has met with hundreds of decision makers, including kings, presidents, prime ministers, ministers of health and finance as well as people affected by leprosy, whose communities he has made a point of visiting.

Besides his physical presence, or words of encouragement and concrete support for local services, Mr. Sasakawa was proactive enough to propose and discuss new initiatives and strategies with the leprosy community to guarantee the maintenance and development of each country's anti-leprosy measures, and make stakeholders aware of the need for further efforts during the post-elimination era. This aspect of his agenda is discussed below.

Contributing with new strategies—leprosy as a human rights issue

At the end of the year 2000, the global prevalence rate was just below one case per 10,000 population, enabling WHO and its partners to announce in 2001 that the overall target set ten years earlier for the global elimination of leprosy as a public health problem had been reached. However, back in June 1998, the WHO indicated for the first time that "some countries may need to continue and intensify activities beyond the year 2000 to reach their elimination targets". In view of this, WHO recommended that a long-term comprehensive strategy for leprosy be developed; this appeared as The final push towards elimination of leprosy: strategic plan 2000–2005 (2000). This was just the first additional initiative to enhance the strategy, since many others followed "the final push": the Global strategy for further reducing the leprosy burden and sustaining leprosy control activities (2006–2010), the Enhanced global strategy for further reducing the disease burden due to leprosy (2011–2015), the Global Leprosy Strategy 2016–2020: Accelerating towards a leprosy-free world, and Towards Zero Leprosy: Global Leprosy (Hansen's disease) Strategy 2021–2030.

It was an astute decision, since the complex task of eliminating a disease in a diverse group of countries would certainly not pro-

Figure 2: The WHO Global Leprosy Strategy 2016–2020

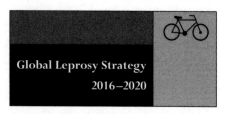

ceed at an even pace in each of them. Therefore these additional enhancements were proposed in timely fashion at specific moments when the interim analysis of the results showed extra efforts were needed to assure the continuity of the elimination process. Among these enhancements I should like to call special attention to the Global Leprosy Strategy for 2016–20, with its tagline "Accelerating towards a leprosy-free world".

The strategy has a central message conveyed by the image of a bicycle (Figure 2), iconography that is closely linked to the Ambassador's habit of talking about leprosy in terms of a motorcycle, where "The front wheel represents our efforts to tackle the disease, and the back wheel our fight against stigma and discrimination. Unless both wheels turn at the same time, it will not be possible to eliminate leprosy from the world."[15]

Mr. Sasakawa hit on this idea after watching The Motorcycle Diaries, a movie depicting the epic journey through Latin America of the Argentinian revolutionary Che Guevara, who visits a leprosarium in a remote area of Peru, volunteering his services as a doctor. From this, we understand that the medical and social aspects of leprosy have the same relevance and must be addressed together.

The front wheel of the motorcycle, the medical one, seems to have been gathering speed in recent years, with plenty of great achievements in the elimination of the disease. However, the back wheel, the social aspects of leprosy, has been neglected. People affected by leprosy still face serious issues with regards to stigma and discrimination. In other words, although the front wheel has been spinning in the right direction, the back wheel has been holding up progress. Therefore the "motorcycle" needs some fine-tuning. The WHO strategy for 2016–20, using the symbol of a bicycle, no doubt inspired by Mr. Sasakawa's motorcycle, was an opportunity to adjust the back wheel in such a way that the bicycle can move ahead and accelerate to a world free of leprosy.

With this aim, the new strategy was structured around three pillars: 1) strengthen government ownership, coordination and partnership; 2) stop leprosy and its complications; and 3) stop discrimination and promote inclusion.

In addition to the focus on the "back wheel" represented by the third pillar, the strategy also had some specific interim targets that would have an impact on the social consequences for leprosy: 1) zero disability among new child cases; 2) reduction of visible disabilities among new cases to less than one per million population; and 3) zero countries with legislation allowing discrimination on the basis of leprosy. Given the Ambassador's close involvement in the fight against discrimination of persons affected by leprosy, this strategy was in line with his increasing focus on ending the discrimination faced by persons affected by leprosy.

The first time he spoke out about human rights issues around leprosy was at the Forum 2000 Conference in 2001, in a keynote address on "The Human Right to Health". The Forum, founded in 1997, was an initiative of Václav Havel, former president of the Czech Republic; Elie Wiesel, a survivor of Auschwitz and Nobel Prize recipient; and Mr. Yohei Sasakawa himself. The Forum was to serve as a platform for global dialogue pursuing the path towards world peace, for the sake of the future of all humanity.

In the early 2000s, Mr. Sasakawa endeavoured to make the Office of the United Nations High Commissioner for Human Rights aware of the need to address discrimination in leprosy as a human rights issue—and he succeeded. Later, he was able to attend the 60th session of the United Nations Commission on Human Rights (UNCHR) where, for the first time, he addressed members of the Commission on the discrimination faced by persons affected by leprosy. This was a turning point in making decision makers aware that leprosy is an issue that goes beyond purely medical concerns and must be handled together with its social aspects. Indeed, Mr. Sasakawa pointed out something that was somewhat absent from the perspective of medical personnel and scientists; namely, that the fear of stigma remains a major barrier to early diagnosis and treatment and thus hampers the interruption of transmission.

Ultimately, the strong message of Mr. Sasakawa was that the disease will be defeated only when "the number of people who discriminate against people affected by the disease also diminishes".[16] This was soon recognized by the WHO, which for the first time added assignments on eliminating stigma and discrimination to his mandate as WHO Goodwill Ambassador. As Mr. Sasakawa himself has mentioned in his newsletter, the significance of this resides in the fact that it meant that the WHO was thinking about leprosy not only in a medical context but in a social context, too. Indeed, it is essential that the two go hand in hand. To engage the United Nations Human Rights Council, and to involve society at large, the WHO, governments, NGOs and people affected by leprosy themselves must work together for this purpose.

A sound example of Mr. Sasakawa's commitment to human rights is his strategy to empower leprosy-affected persons to stand up for their rights, given that the authorities do not appear particularly concerned on their behalf. In many documents, in formal speeches and through practical actions, the Ambassador has made clear that leprosy-affected persons must be the main actors in the fight against the disease and the discrimination they face. Practical actions are those where, in his capacity as WHO Goodwill Ambassador, Mr. Sasakawa has provided the opportunity for leprosy-affected persons to directly interact with political leaders and voice their needs and demands.

For instance, this strategy was successful in Brazil when he visited the country in 2004 and met then President Luiz Inácio Lula da Silva. The Ambassador, in a straightforward speech, called on the government to make greater efforts for leprosy elimination. The president, recognizing the grave situation, was humble and pragmatic in his reply to Mr. Sasakawa: "We could have solved this problem of leprosy long before, but we did not try hard enough. We need to make up for lost time."[17] Indeed, this was the start of a new strategy to address the leprosy burden and fight discrimination against affected persons.

The president was quite impressed by the resolve of Mr. Sasakawa. A further result of this first contact was the participation of President Lula da Silva as a signatory to Mr. Sasakawa's first annual Global Appeal to end stigma and discrimination against persons affected by leprosy in 2006, together with former US President Jimmy Carter and the Dalai Lama, among others. Another example of this strategy was his successful visit to Brazil in 2019, where he was received by President Bolsonaro. Visiting Maranhão, a state in northern Brazil with a high leprosy burden, Mr. Sasakawa was able to gather together in the same room the State Governor, local authorities, health personnel and leprosy-affected persons for a substantive and productive conference on the social determinants of the disease. This was a key opportunity to allow affected persons to voice their needs and learn how to make their rights a reality.

Mr. Sasakawa's commitment to promoting human rights is evidenced by the annual Global Appeal, which shows his capacity to mobilize the support of respected individuals and organizations from diverse fields and have them lend their voices to ending the stigma and discrimination that persons affected by leprosy face. In so doing, he has increased awareness of this issue in spaces that were previously silent about it.

Leprosy control in the post-elimination era

The WHO elimination strategy, based on the widespread coverage of MDT and also on the concept of what constitutes a cured leprosy case, was focused on reducing prevalence. After a while, it was clear that the prevalence rate was not the best measure of the elimination target, and the focus changed to the new case detection rate (reducing incidence), disability, and stigma and discrimination.

These advances, together with the recent adoption of a single dose of rifampicin as chemoprophylaxis for contacts of leprosy cases, have encouraged the WHO to review the leprosy elimination target, now defined as no new autochthonous cases as a result of interruption of transmission. Based on this, an updated concept of elimination was introduced. According to the latest WHO road map for neglected tropical diseases, elimination (interruption of transmission) means a reduction to zero of the incidence of infection caused by a specific pathogen in a defined geographical area, with minimal risk of reintroduction, as a result of deliberate efforts; continued action to prevent re-establishment of transmission may be required.[18]

In fact, since 2018 there is a new scenario for the fight against leprosy and a more realistic view of a leprosy-free world, with a new approach to achieve it—the "zero leprosy" strategy. The aim of zero leprosy is straightforward: to end leprosy. It has a triple vision: no disease, no disability and no discrimination. Although its vision is clear, zero leprosy is also a daunting task. However, the tenacity and the willingness of stakeholders and health personnel to take on this new challenge suggests it is something within reach. To make this vision appealing and feasible, a Global Partnership for Zero Leprosy (GPZL) was launched in January 2018.

GPZL is a coalition of organizations and individuals committed to ending leprosy. The partnership includes Novartis, the WHO—as an observer—the International Federation of Anti-Leprosy Associations (ILEP), the Sasakawa Health Foundation (SHF) and the International Association for Integration, Dignity and Economic Advancement (IDEA). It also includes representatives from the national leprosy programmes of Brazil, Ghana and India, the International Leprosy Association (ILA), scientific organizations and the academic community.

GPZL aims at providing technical support (road maps, action plans) as well as suggesting and stimulating the conduct of research in key areas to support countries to achieve zero leprosy. The advantages of having such a coalition are manifold: 1) it is a private-sector initiative, which assures it some freedom of movement; 2) it is very well received by the leprosy community, since all major members of this community feel represented within the coalition; 3) GPZL offers high-quality technical guidance to governments aiming for zero leprosy as a political achievement; and 4), most importantly, persons affected by leprosy are actively involved in GPZL. In addition, the framework in which GPZL was designed favours the active involvement of participants in various areas such as project implementation, research, policymaking, fundraising and advocacy, which, in brief, are the core initiatives for a successful partnership.

Ultimately, GPZL acts as a proactive platform to get the zero leprosy strategy running, initially based on the following three pillars, mirroring the WHO's 2016–2020 Global Leprosy Strategy: 1) Strengthen government ownership, coordination and partnership; 2) Stop leprosy and its complications; 3) Stop discrimination and promote inclusion.

Although not Mr. Sasakawa's idea, it is worth noting that each of the GPZL pillars relates closely to both the Ambassador's philosophy and his actions. His continuous visits to authorities, field workers and persons affected by leprosy convey a constant message to strengthen their participation in the fight against leprosy, stimulating government ownership, optimizing coordination of actions and promoting partnership at various levels. His awareness that training health personnel was a priority task to attain leprosy elimination has been seen in his effective support for training and capacity-building activities through the BDSF and other means, and is a simple but pivotal contribution of the Ambassador towards the goal of ending leprosy and its complications.

Lastly, concerning the third pillar, it is worth mentioning that in 2016, the Ambassador was able to organize, together with the Pontifical Council for Health Care Workers and the Good Samaritan Foundation, a memorable meeting in the Vatican to discuss and share best practices to improve access to medical treatment and to protect those with leprosy from exclusion and isolation. The meeting, which brought together representatives of the three main world religions, medical experts, scientists, health workers and persons affected by leprosy, concluded that "the elimination of the stigma attached to leprosy requires an important work of education that must involve all social groups and in particular religious communities because they promote respect for human dignity throughout the world".

In this sense, the meeting was instrumental in enlisting the support of prominent religious leaders in teaching their followers correct concepts about leprosy and dispelling many discriminatory beliefs attached to the disease and those it affects. Although a sophisticated medical and technical meeting, the hidden agenda, so to speak, of many of the speeches and presentations centred on having compassion for people who are suffering a double scourge— an infectious disease and a stigmatizing condition. The success of the meeting and its agenda was not the result of chance: the outcome was carefully conceived. It was a clear example of why Mr. Sasakawa's mandate as WHO Goodwill Ambassador for Leprosy Elimination remains relevant in a post-elimination era, and why a Goodwill Ambassador is still needed.

The fact remains that leprosy still exists, and we must not forget it. This relates closely to the third part of the Ambassador's philosophy: "I must keep going until results are obtained."

Despite the striking positive modification on the epidemiologic data on leprosy, there are still many people affected by leprosy in many countries. Truly, the last mile to a world free of leprosy is a long one. Thus, there is a new role in the post-elimination era for the WHO Goodwill Ambassador: to be the Goodwill Ambassador for a World Free of Leprosy. He has the experience, the leadership and the proactiveness to assume this role.

Actually, he recognizes this in the statement quoted above, which he makes concrete while translating words into action through his many deeds. Examples of this are his campaign launched in 2021 aimed at stakeholders called "Don't Forget Leprosy", and his declaration, in 2015, that "an increase in patient numbers is not something to be ashamed of; it should be commended as a sign of an active program". It is encouraging to hear the Ambassador declare: "There are still people suffering from leprosy in places we don't know about; there are still leprosy hot spots. Let us go all out and find these new cases."[19] This is what we need to control leprosy in the post-elimination era, and Mr. Sasakawa can be the guiding light to illuminate the way, as he has been so far.

Guidance is still needed to go for the triple targets of zero leprosy by detecting new cases through control activities, as recommended by the WHO. Improvement in drug regimens for treatment may be opportune, as well as chemoprophylaxis to interrupt the transmission of the disease. However, despite the advances in science and technology, we still know little about the transmission of Mycobacterium leprae, the role of animal reservoirs, and the course of the infection.

In this sense, the post-elimination era must be based on a three-point agenda: continued efforts to make sure that quality leprosy services are available to the communities in need (including training of health personnel and regular supply of free MDT); effective measures to eliminate stigma and discrimination; and robust research into the mechanisms of leprosy transmission that can be translated into strategies to interrupt transmission.

In this connection, the Ambassador has made his mandate fruitful through his continued efforts to stimulate the WHO to provide a clear post-elimination strategy that addresses these three points. These efforts were visible through the launch in 2018 of the WHO Guidelines for the Diagnosis, Treatment and Prevention of Leprosy. The careful production of this text followed strictly the WHO's GRADE approach, in which all available evidence published in English was taken into consideration. Funding support was provided by TNF and the result is a fine volume addressing state-of-the-art knowledge and evidence on leprosy. Other examples of the strategy are the adoption of single-dose rifampicin as a pre-exposure prophylaxis (SDR-PEP) and the introduction of new criteria for elimination of leprosy.

The COVID-19 pandemic has taught us that humans are fragile organisms vulnerable to new viruses in the environment, despite the striking advances in health science and technology. SARS-CoV-2 spread rapidly worldwide, with 767 million confirmed cases and over 6.9 million deaths as of July 12, 2023.

By contrast, leprosy is an old problem we have been grappling with for centuries. However, presently it is still a hazard in some countries. For that, the Ambassador should strengthen his position as a facilitator of the journey along the last but longest mile to free the world from leprosy, based on his second philosophical principle: taking action to transform society requires a strong and committed spirit that can withstand hardships.

Yes, he can push on with public information campaigns to change traditionally negative perceptions of leprosy, to address the issues of stigma and discrimination, to convince low- and high-ranking authorities to amend or abolish discriminatory laws, to support measures aiming to maintain and strengthen capacity for clinical diagnosis, or research to develop a point-of-care test to confirm diagnosis and detect infection in populations at risk and, especially, to support studies to develop a vaccine to improve prevention of new leprosy cases. All these topics are included in the three-point agenda for the post-elimination era noted above: continued efforts to make sure that quality leprosy services are available to the communities in need (including training of health personnel and regular supply of free MDT); effective measures to eliminate stigma and discrimination; and robust research into the mechanisms of leprosy transmission that can be translated into strategies to interrupt transmission.

However, most of all, he must be a humble preacher of compassion, because, as Rousseau stated, compassion, which is a natural human impulse, is a useful manifestation of the otherwise dangerous desire to extend the self and to show signs of power. Compassion allows man to experience this relationality, transporting him towards others as he identifies with their suffering, recalling the finitude and vulnerability shared by all creatures.

Mr. Yohei Sasakawa's role as Goodwill Ambassador has been pivotal in sustaining political commitment in endemic countries he has visited, some of them many times. His emphasis on empowerment of leprosy-affected people and protecting their human rights through fighting stigma and discrimination has been invaluable. Ultimately, an ambassador is a politician and we expect him to act as such. Interestingly, Mr. Sasakawa differs from a typical ambassador because he goes far beyond that description. He is not just a person of words and gestures: he is a man of action. He identifies a problem, he proposes a solution and actually promotes effective action to solve the problem. He is attentive to the latest scientific achievements on leprosy, concerned for the effective provision of drugs for treating the disease, keen to support the training of technical personnel and unequivocally requests that persons affected by leprosy are assured of their human rights.

While the results of his mandate can be measured in the number of trips and speeches, encounters and meetings he has carried out, this would give only a faint idea of the real changes he provokes among those with whom he interacts. It is also difficult to measure the effectiveness of his actions through crude epidemiological figures or medical statistics, since his interventions are not directly technical. He exceeds what is expected of a Goodwill Ambassador, giving more than is expected of him, while the results he wants to achieve do not give him any personal gain, but are fully appropriated by the community.

It is impossible to quantify the joy and hope Mr. Sasakawa brings to leprosy-affected persons, the inspiration he instils in health workers, leading to their renewed commitment, and, finally, the awareness he prompts in politicians on the medical, social and political relevance of leprosy. In brief, he acts similarly to the tide, which comes and goes in ceaseless motion. Flowing, he generously fills the needs of those lacking awareness and hope. Then back, with a strong majestic sweep he rolls in ebb to renew, tirelessly, his and others' commitment.

Over the course of his mandate, this is the concrete evidence of the effectiveness of Mr. Sasakawa's work, and a testimony for him to continue on the same path till the end of the last and longest mile to a world free of leprosy.

NOTES

1. TOWARDS A LEPROSY-FREE WORLD: THE PIONEERING ACTIVITIES OF MR. YOHEI SASAKAWA

1. In 2007, the government of Japan decided to make "appealing to international society for the elimination of discrimination related to leprosy" a pillar of its diplomacy, and in 2009 reappointed Mr. Yohei Sasakawa as its Goodwill Ambassador for the Human Rights of Persons Affected by Leprosy. https://www.mofa.go.jp/announce/event/2009/4/1190316_1156.html (accessed 9 December 2021).

2. "WHO Goodwill Ambassador for Leprosy Elimination's role is to make sure that leprosy is not forgotten", *WHO Goodwill Ambassador's Leprosy Bulletin*, no. 104, July 2021, p. 2.

3. "Yohei Sasakawa Receives WHO Medal", The Nippon Foundation, 28 April 2017. https://www.nippon-foundation.or.jp/en/news/articles/2017/20 170428-21168.html (accessed 9 December 2021).

4. https://www.in.emb-japan.go.jp/itpr_en/00_000807.html (accessed 9 December 2021).

5. In regard to the history of leprosy, see Shigeki Sakamoto, "Draft of principles and guidelines on elimination of discrimination against persons affected by leprosy and their family members" (A/HRC/AC/3/CRP.2), pp. 6–8, paras. 14–26.

6. Yohei Sasakawa, *No Matter Where the Journey Takes Me: One Man's Quest for a Leprosy-Free World* (London: Hurst, 2019), p. 5.

7. *Ibid.*, p. 8.

8. UN General Assembly, Work of the Statistical Commission pertaining to the 2030 Agenda for Sustainable Development (A/RES/71/313). The specific indicators are listed in the Annex of the Resolution.

9. UN General Assembly, Transforming our world: the 2030 Agenda for Sustainable Development (A/RES/70/1), p. 2.

10. Sasakawa, *No Matter Where the Journey Takes Me*, p. 7.

11. From 2000 to the present, the free provision of MDT continues to be carried out through Novartis/the Novartis Foundation. According to Novartis, currently from 2 to 3 million people are living with physical disability and stigma as a result of leprosy. "Leprosy", https://www.novartis.com/diseases/leprosy (accessed 10 December 2021).

12. Fumihiko Takayama, *The Last and Longest Mile: Yohei Sasakawa's Struggle to Eliminate Leprosy* (London: Hurst, 2021), pp. 65–86.

13. Statement on the second meeting of the International Health Regulations (2005) Emergency Committee regarding the outbreak of novel coronavirus (2019-nCoV), 30 January 2020. https://www.who.int/news/item/30-01-2020-statement-on-the-second-meeting-of-the-international-health-regulations-(2005)-emergency-committee-regarding-the-outbreak-of-novel-coronavirus-(2019-nCoV) (accessed 10 December 2021).

14. António Guterres, "We are all in this Together: Human Rights and COVID-19 Response and Recovery", 23 April 2020. https://www.un.org/en/un-coronavirus-communications-teams/we-are-all-together-human-rights-and-covid-19-response-and-recovery (accessed 10 December 2021).

15. "WHO Director-General's opening remarks at the media briefing on COVID-19—29 June 2020". https//www.who.int/director-general/speeches/detail/who-director-general-s-opening-remarks-at-the-media-briefing-on-covid-19-29-june-2020 (accessed 10 December 2021).

16. António Guterres, "UN chief: COVID-19 vaccine must be affordable and available to all", https://news.un.org/en/story/2020/09/1072522 (accessed 10 December 2021).

17. "The rights and health of refugees, migrants and stateless must be protected in COVID-19 response", https://www.unhcr.org/news/news-releases/rights-and-health-refugees-migrants-and-stateless-must-be-protected-covid-19 (accessed 10 December 2021).

18. 44th Session of the Human Rights Council, Global update on human rights and the impact of the COVID-19 pandemic: Statement by Michelle Bachelet, UN High Commissioner for Human Rights, 30 June 2020. https//www.ohchr.org/en/statements/2020/06/44th-session-human-rights-councilglobal-update-human-rights-and-impact-covid-19 (accessed 21 June 2023).

19. "No exceptions with COVID-19: 'Everyone has the right to life-saving interventions'—UN experts say", 26 March 2020. https://www.ohchr.org/EN/NewsEvents/Pages/DisplayNews.aspx?NewsID=25746&LangID=E (accessed 10 December 2021).

20. However, it is important to remember that infectious disease measures risk relativizing the value of an individual life when viewed in relation to the safety of society as a whole. With the medical breakdown caused by the COVID-19 pandemic, the issue of the intensive triage that took place in Italy leads to difficult problems from the viewpoint of respect for the right to life of the individual.

21. It is difficult to cultivate the causative bacteria for leprosy, and since, apart from

human beings, the disease affects only very few animals such as armadillos, development is difficult. However, Dr. Jacinto Convit of Venezuela developed a vaccine using armadillos. On 8 December 1987, Mr. Ryoichi Sasakawa, father of Yohei, received the first leprosy vaccination at the WHO Headquarters in Geneva. See "Working for a World without Leprosy", The Nippon Foundation, 2020, p. 25.

22. *Ibid.*, p. 16.

23. *Ibid.*, p. 19.

24. *Ibid.*, p. 21.

25. WHO Study Group, "Chemotherapy of leprosy for control programmes: report of a WHO study group [meeting held in Geneva from 12 to 16 October 1981]" (WHO, 1982). https://apps.who.int/iris/handle/10665/38984 (accessed 20 December 2021).

26. Cairns S. Smith *et al.*, "Multidrug therapy for leprosy: a game changer on the path to elimination", *The Lancet. Infectious Diseases* 17(9) (2017), e294. Published Online, 7 July 2017, https://pubmed.ncbi.nlm.nih.gov/28693853/ (accessed 20 December 2021).

27. WHO Study Group, "Chemotherapy of leprosy for control programmes (1982).

28. Smith *et al.*, "Multidrug therapy for leprosy", e293.

29. 44th World Health Assembly, "Leprosy", 13 May 1991 (WHA44.9), para.1.

30. *Ibid.*, Endnotes, note 1.

31. It is considered that Dr. S. K. Noordeen, then the head of the WHO's Global Leprosy Unit, and Dr. Yo Yuasa of the Sasakawa Health Foundation, who was involved in a similar initiative in the WHO's Western Pacific Region, were key proponents of this unique approach to public health activities. "Working for a World without Leprosy" (2020), p. 26.

32. In regard to a discussion on the times when this kind of goal-setting is an appropriate means of control, and on the conditions required for a goal-oriented agenda to bring about beneficial results, see Norichika Kanie and Frank Bierman, eds., *Governing through Goals: Sustainable Development Goals as Governance Innovation* (Cambridge, MA: MIT Press, 2017).

33. *Working for a World without Leprosy* (2020), p. 27. As a result, Egypt and Mexico (1994), Thailand and Sri Lanka (1995), Colombia (1996), Benin, Venezuela and Chad (1997), etc., countries that had still not conquered leprosy, all successively achieved its elimination as a public health problem. The year in brackets shows when this was achieved. The concepts of elimination and eradication differ fundamentally. Further, there is insufficient surveillance in some developing countries, and problems with statistics, while issues related to providing care for persons affected by leprosy who have persisting disability remain. See Diana N. J. Lockwood and Sujai Suneetha, "Leprosy: too complex a disease for a simple elimination paradigm", *Bulletin of the World Health Organization* 83(3) (March 2005), pp. 230–5. https://apps.who.int/iris/bitstream/handle/10665/269365/PMC2624210.pdf?sequence=1&isAllowed=y (accessed 28 December 2021).

34. According to this, the scale of MDT provision expanded from 38% in 1992 to 99.2% in 2000. Statement by Dr. Hussein A. Gezairy, Regional Director WHO Eastern Mediterranean Region to the First Meeting of Global Alliance for Elimination of Leprosy, New Delhi, India, 30–31 January 2001, p. 2. https://apps.who.int/iris/bitstream/handle/10665/125771/message_First%20meeting%20_alliance%20_New%20Delhi_2001_en.pdf?sequence=1&isAllowed=y (accessed 12 December 2021).

35. "WHO in action: eliminating leprosy; Hanoi Declaration calls for stronger commitment", *World Health* 47(5) (1994), p. 1. https://apps.who.int/iris/handle/10665/328647 (accessed 7 December 2021).

36. "Working for a World without Leprosy" (2020), p. 27.

37. However, there are many so-called hot spots of the disease in leprosy-endemic countries where prevalence of the disease is high and access is difficult, and some estimates put the number of hidden cases as high as 3 million.

38. There was criticism of WHO for calling the campaign involving GAEL the "Final Push" against leprosy. See Kommer L. Braber, "An evaluation of GAEL, the Global Alliance for the Elimination of Leprosy", *Leprosy Review* 75(3) (2004), pp. 210–12.

39. Novartis promises to provide MDT drugs free of charge until at least 2025. WHO, "Leprosy", 27 January 2023, https://www.who.int/news-room/fact-sheets/detail/leprosy (accessed 17 July 2023).

40. "First Meeting of the Global Alliance for Elimination of Leprosy—GAEL", New Delhi, India, 20 and 31 January 2001 (WHO/CDS/CPE/CEE/2001.27), p. 43, Annex 4, "The Delhi Declaration". https://apps.who.int/iris/bitstream/handle/10665/66944/WHO_CDS_CPE_CEE_2001.27.pdf?sequence=1&isAllowed=y (accessed 11 December 2021).

41. For details, see "Leprosy in Our Time", The Nippon Foundation, November 2014, p. 6. https://www.nippon-foundation.or.jp/app/uploads/2019/01/Leprosy_in_Our_Time2014.pdf (accessed 11 December 2021).

42. "Working for a World without Leprosy" (2020), p. 33.

43. "Consultative relationship between the United Nations and non-governmental organizations", Resolution 1996/31, 49th plenary meeting, 25 July 1996, ECOSOC.

44. "Discrimination against leprosy victims and their families", UN Sub-Commission on the Promotion and Protection of Human Rights, Resolution 2004/12.

45. José Bengoa, Yozo Yokota *et al.*, "Discrimination against leprosy victims and their families: draft resolution", E/CN.4/Sub.2/2005/L.37, 17 October 2005, p. 3, para. 10.

46. Yozo Yokota, "Preliminary working paper on discrimination against leprosy victims and their families", E/CN.4/Sub.2/2005/WP.1, 14 July 2005, p. 5, para. 13. The following year, in August 2006, Mr. Yokota provided a "Preliminary report on discrimination against leprosy affected persons and their families" to the Sub-Commission on Prevention of Discrimination and Protection of Minorities (A/HRC/Sub.1/58/CRP.7).

47. Human Rights Council, Resolution 8/13, Elimination of discrimination against persons affected by leprosy and their family members (A/HRC/RES/8/13), paras.1, 3 and 5.

48. Report of the Advisory Committee on its first session, Geneva, 4–15 August 2008 (A/HRC/AC/2008/1/2), p. 15.

49. Report of the United Nations High Commissioner for Human Rights and Report of the Office of the High Commissioner and the Secretary-General: Report of the elimination of discrimination against persons affected by leprosy and their family members (A/HRC/10/62), pp. 13–19, paras. 30–37.

50. Working Paper on the Elimination of discrimination against persons affected by leprosy and their family members (A/HRC/AC/2/CRP.5), paras.20–21.

51. For more details on the contents of the Principles and Guidelines, see Principles and Guidelines on Elimination of discrimination against persons affected by leprosy and their family members (A/HRC/15/30, Annex).

52. UNHRC Resolution 15/10. Elimination of discrimination against persons affected by leprosy and their family members (A/HRC/RES/15/10), p. 1, para. 1.

53. UNHRC Resolution 65/215. Elimination of discrimination against persons affected by leprosy and their family members (A/HRC/RES/65/215), p. 1, paras. 1–2.

54. "Working for a World without Leprosy" (2020), p. 44.

55. UNHRC, Resolution 29/5. Elimination of discrimination against persons affected by leprosy and their family members (A/HRC/RES/29/5), p. 2, paras. 1–2.

56. Preliminary Report on the implementation of the principles and guidelines for the elimination of discrimination against persons affected by leprosy and their family members prepared by Imeru Tamrat Yigezu (A/HRC/AC/16/CPR.2), p. 4, para. 9.

57. Progress Report on the implementation of the principles and guidelines for the elimination of discrimination against persons affected by leprosy and their family members prepared by Imeru Tamrat Yigezu (A/HRC/AC/17/CPR.1), pp. 21–2, para. 80; p. 23, para. 86.

58. Resolution 35/9 adopted by the Human Rights Council on 22 June 2017 (A/HRC/RES/35/9), pp. 2–3, para. 1.

59. https://www.ohchr.org/EN/Issues/Leprosy/Pages/LeprosyIndex.aspx (accessed 20 December 2021) and Yohei Sasakawa, "My Hopes for the Special Rapporteur", WHO Goodwill Ambassador's Newsletter, no. 87, October 2017, p. 1.

60. Resolution 44/6 adopted by the Human Rights Council on 16 July 2020 (A/HRC/RES/44/6), p. 2, para. 2

61. Stigmatization as dehumanization: wrongful stereotyping and structural violence against women and children affected by leprosy (A/HRC/41/47).

62. Visit to Brazil, Report of the Special Rapporteur on the elimination of discrimination against persons affected by leprosy and their family members (A/

HRC/44/46/Add. 2); Visit to Japan, Report of the Special Rapporteur on the elimination of discrimination against persons affected by leprosy and their family members (A/HRC/44/46/Add.1).

63. Elimination of discrimination against persons affected by leprosy and their family members: Note by the Secretary-General (A/76/148), pp. 1–22 (accessed 27 December 2021).

64. Yohei Sasakawa, "After the Summit", *WHO Goodwill Ambassador's Newsletter*, no. 63, August 2013, p. 1.

65. "Bangkok Declaration: Towards a Leprosy-free World", pp. 3–4, paras. 1–2. https://www.afro.who.int/sites/default/files/2017–06/bangkok_declaration.pdf (accessed 8 December 2021).

66. One example of these preservation efforts is the Culion Museum and Archives. Culion Island in the Philippines was once a leprosy colony and the Museum and Archives preserves this history. The Museum and Archives was officially inscribed in the UNESCO Memory of the World Register—Asia and the Pacific Region in 2018.

2. ELIMINATION OF LEPROSY AS A PUBLIC HEALTH PROBLEM

1. H. Sansarricq, ed., *Multidrug therapy against leprosy: Development and implementation over the past 25 years* (World Health Organization, 2004), pp. 145–6.

2. Brian H. Bennett, MD, MPH, David L. Parker, MD, MPH, and Mark Robson, PhD, MPH, "Leprosy: steps along the journey of eradication", Public Health Rep. 2008 Mar–Apr; 123(2): 198–205.doi: 10.1177/003335490812300212; PMC2239329;PMID: 18457072.

3. David J. Blok, Sake J. De Vlas and Jan Hendrick Richardus, "Global elimination of leprosy by 2020: are we on track?", *Parasites & Vectors* 8 (548) (2015). https://doi.org/10.1186/s13071–015–1143–4 (accessed 2 July 2023).

3. LEPROSY AS A HUMAN RIGHTS ISSUE

1. Universal Declaration of Human Rights, https://www.ohchr.org/EN/UDHR/Pages/Language.aspx?LangID (accessed 27 December 2021).

2. The Japan Shipbuilding Industry Foundation, later to become the Nippon Foundation, was established in 1962. From the start, it expended efforts in constructing buildings connected with leprosy hospitals in various countries in Asia. In 1974, in order to focus more strongly on global leprosy elimination, it created the Sasakawa Memorial Health Foundation (known since 2019 as Sasakawa Health Foundation), with Professor Morizo Ishidate of Tokyo University, who had been the first person in Japan to successfully synthesize the leprosy drug promin (sodium glucosulfone), as its first chair.

3. In 2001, Mr. Sasakawa was appointed as the Special Ambassador of the Global Alliance for the Elimination of Leprosy (GAEL), a group established by the

WHO, national governments and NGOs. Subsequently, after GAEL was disbanded, in 2004 he was appointed as the WHO Goodwill Ambassador for Leprosy Elimination, a position he holds to this day.

4. From an interview with Mr. Sasakawa on 24 August 2021.

5. Forum 2000 is an annual international conference that was begun at the suggestion of three people: Mr. Václav Havel, former president of the Czech Republic; Mr. Elie Wiesel, a writer and Nobel Peace Prize recipient; and Mr. Sasakawa, with the objective of discussing and resolving issues of mutual concern to all of humanity. The first conference was held in Prague, Czech Republic.

6. Yohei Sasakawa, *Making the Impossible Possible: My Work for Leprosy Elimination and Human Rights* (London: Hurst, 2023), p. 58.

7. The WHO, at the 44th World Health Assembly held in May 1991, adopted a resolution to eliminate leprosy as a public health problem (defined as a reduction in prevalence to less than one registered patient per 10,000 population). This goal was achieved at the global level by the end of 2000, leaving only fourteen countries yet to reach that milestone at the national level. GAEL, mentioned above, was established to realize elimination in these high-burden countries.

8. The Sub-Commission had the equivalent function of the current Human Rights Council Advisory Committee, but unlike the latter had the authority to adopt its own resolutions and to make recommendations to the Commission on Human Rights.

9. "Good News on Human Rights", *WHO Goodwill Ambassador's Newsletter*, no. 16, October 2005, p. 2.

10. The UN, in order to strengthen its ability to respond to human rights issues, replaced the UN Commission on Human Rights, which had been established by the Economic and Social Council (ECOSOC), with the UN Human Rights Council, which is an auxiliary organization of the UN General Assembly. The Human Rights Council is made up of 47 members states (down from 53 in the days of the Commission) who serve for three years and are not eligible for immediate re-election after serving two consecutive terms. Council members are elected by direct and secret ballot by members of the UN General Assembly, unlike Commission members who were elected by ECOSOC, and the Council is thus directly accountable to all UN member states.

11. Resolution adopted by Human Rights Council on 18 June 2008 (A/HRC/RES/8/13).

12. Sasakawa, *Making the Impossible Possible*, p. 38.

13. Resolution adopted by Human Rights Council on 12 October 2009 (A/HRC/RES/12/7).

14. Resolution adopted by Human Rights Council on 6 October 2010 (A/HRC/RES/15/10).

15. Resolution adopted by Human Rights Council on 12 August 2010 (A/HRC/RES/15/30).

16. Yohei Sasakawa, *No Matter Where the Journey Takes Me: One Man's Quest for a Leprosy-Free World* (London: Hurst, 2019), p. 17.

17. Shigeki Sakamoto, "Principles and guidelines for the elimination of stigma and discrimination against persons affected by leprosy and their family members", *Kansai University Review of Law and Politics* (in Japanese) 61(3) (Faculty of Law, Kansai University, 2011), pp. 754–805.

18. Yozo Yokota, "Global movement to fight against discrimination", *Leprosy: Japan and the World* [translated from Japanese] (Tokyo: Kosakusha, 2016), pp. 276–82.

19. International Working Group on Leprosy and Human Rights, *Working Together to Eliminate All Forms of Discrimination Associated with Leprosy*, International Working Group on Leprosy and Human Rights, 2015.

20. Resolution adopted by Human Rights Council on 2 July 2015 (A/HRC/RES/29/5).

21. Progress Report on the Implementation of the principles and guidelines for the elimination of discrimination against persons affected by leprosy and their family members (A/HRC/AC/17/CRP.1).

22. A survey by the Sasakawa-India Leprosy Foundation (S-ILF) found that there were 758 colonies in India (as of March 2020).

23. Draft report on the implementation of the principles and guidelines for the elimination of discrimination against persons affected by leprosy and their family members (A/HRC/18/CRP.1), p. 21.

24. Resolution adopted by Human Rights Council on 12 July 2017 (A/HRC/RES/35/9).

25. Resolution adopted by Human Rights Council on 22 July 2020 (A/HRC/RES/44/6). At the 53rd session of the Human Rights Council held in July 2023, the term of Special Rapporeur was extended for three years again.

26. From an interview with Mr. Sasakawa on 24 August 2021.

27. Up until December 2021, the Nippon Foundation and the Sasakawa Health Foundation have provided support to 32 groups of persons affected by leprosy in 19 countries (see Chapter 4 in this volume).

28. Report of the Special Rapporteur on the elimination of discrimination against persons affected by leprosy and their family members (A/HRC/38/42).

29. Stigmatization as dehumanization: wrongful stereotyping and structural violence against women and children affected by leprosy—Report of the Special Rapporteur on the elimination of discrimination against persons affected by leprosy and their family members (A/HRC/41/47).

30. Policy framework for rights-based action plans—Report of the Special Rapporteur on the elimination of discrimination against persons affected by leprosy and their family members (A/HRC/44/46).

31. Disproportionate impact of the coronavirus disease (COVID-19) pandemic on persons affected by leprosy and their family members: root causes, consequences and the way to recovery—Report of the Special Rapporteur on the elimination

of discrimination against persons affected by leprosy and their family members (A/HRC/47/29).

32. Right to the highest attainable standard of physical and mental health for persons affected by leprosy and their family members—Report of the Special Rapporteur on the elimination of discrimination against persons affected by leprosy and their family members (A/HRC/50/35).

33. Visit to Brazil—Report of the Special Rapporteur on the elimination of discrimination against persons affected by leprosy and their family members (A/HRC/44/46/Add.2).

34. Visit to Japan—Report of the Special Rapporteur on the elimination of discrimination against persons affected by leprosy and their family members (A/HRC/44/46/Add.1).

35. Report of the Special Rapporteur on the elimination of discrimination against persons affected by leprosy and their family members, "An unfinished business: discrimination in law against persons affected by leprosy and their family members" (A/76/148).

36. Elimination of discrimination against persons affected by leprosy and their family members (A/77/139).

37. ILEP, "Updated list of discriminatory laws", https://ilepfederation.org/updated-list-of-discriminatory-laws/ (accessed 22 February 2023).

38. Law Commission of India, *Eliminating Discrimination Against Persons Affected by Leprosy*, Report No. 256, Government of India, April 2015.

39. Elimination of discrimination against persons affected by leprosy and their family members (A/76/148), pp. 15–16.

40. Takahiro Nanri, "Analysis on Special Allowance Scheme for Persons Affected by Leprosy in India", *Atomi Tourism and Community Studies* [in Japanese] (3) (Faculty of Tourism and Community Studies, Atomi University, 2018), pp. 35–43.

41. Elimination of discrimination against persons affected by leprosy and their family members (A/76/148), p. 15.

42. *Ibid.*, p. 13.

43. World Health Organization, Regional Office for South-East Asia, *Guidelines for strengthening participation of persons affected by leprosy in leprosy services* (New Delhi: World Health Organization, 2011).

44. World Health Organization, Regional Office for South-East Asia, *Global Leprosy Strategy 2016–2020: Accelerating towards a leprosy-free world* (New Delhi: World Health Organization, 2001).

45. World Health Organization, Regional Office for South-East Asia, *Towards Zero Leprosy: Global Leprosy (Hansen's Disease) Strategy 2021–2030* (New Delhi: World Health Organization, 2021).

46. "Summary, Conclusions and Recommendations", Global Forum of People's Organizations on Hansen's Disease, Manila, 7–10 September, 2019, https://www.shf.or.jp/en/information/6813 (accessed 27 December 2021).

47. "My Journey Continues", *WHO Goodwill Ambassador's Newsletter*, no. 100, May 2020, p. 1. https://www.shf.or.jp/wsmhfp/wp-content/uploads/2020/05/11th-202005newsletter100-web.pdf (accessed 27 December 2021).

5. TOWARDS THE EMPOWERMENT OF PERSONS WITH LIVED EXPERIENCE OF LEPROSY

1. Report of the Special Rapporteur on the elimination of discrimination against persons affected by leprosy and their family members (A/HRC/38/42), p. 15.

2. World Health Organization, Regional Office for South-East Asia, *Guidelines for strengthening participation of persons affected by leprosy in leprosy services* (New Delhi: World Health Organization, 2011), p. 13.

3. "You Are the Main Actors", *WHO Goodwill Ambassador's Newsletter*, no. 11, December 2004, p. 1.

4. "People: People who deal with leprosy", https://leprosy.jp/people/yamaguchi/ (accessed 19 March 2022).

5. "IDEA", http://www.idealeprosydignity.org/index.html (accessed 16 March 2022).

6. The total amount of financial support provided by the Nippon Foundation and the Sasakawa Health Foundation to IDEA amounted to 300 million yen (1996–2011). The content of the support activities included strengthening IDEA's base, participation of IDEA parties in international conferences and holding exhibitions at the UN Headquarters.

7. See Chapter 3 in this volume.

8. In regard to the details of the measures taken by Mr. Sasakawa, the Nippon Foundation and the Sasakawa Health Foundation on leprosy and human rights, see Chapter 1 in this volume.

9. *WHO Goodwill Ambassador's Newsletter*, no. 36, February 2009, p. 4.

10. For more details on the Global Appeal, see Chapter 4 in this volume.

11. As a result of the survey re-done by the Sasakawa-India Leprosy Foundation (S-ILF), it was confirmed that as of March 2020, 758 colonies existed in India.

12. *WHO Goodwill Ambassador's Newsletter*, no. 18, February 2006, p. 3.

13. Online meeting with Mr. Vagavathali Narsappa, president of APAL, on 24 March 2022.

14. Rajya Sabha Committee on Petitions Report No. 113 on the "Petition Praying for Integration and Empowerment of Leprosy Affected Persons", p. 7. https://rajyasabha.nic.in/rsnew/Committee_site/Committee_File/ReportFile/8/11/131_2016_6_12.pdf (accessed 23 March 2022).

15. Email interview with Mr. Uday Thakar, APAL adviser, on 16 March 2022.

16. Online meeting with Mr. Vagavathali Narsappa, president of APAL, on 24 March 2022.

17. Yohei Sasakawa, *Making the Impossible Possible: My Work for Leprosy Elimination and Human Rights* (London: Hurst, 2023), p. 286.

18. Interview with Mr. Sasakawa on 15 February 2022.
19. For more details on the Dalai Lama–Sasakawa Scholarship Fund, see Chapter 6 in this volume.
20. Email interview with Mr. Artur Custódio of MORHAN on 18 March 2022.
21. *Ibid.*
22. Information obtained from Brazil's Ministry of Human Rights, through Mr. Artur Custódio, on 18 March 2022.
23. See Chapter 4 in this volume.
24. Email interview with Mr. Al Kadri, vice chairman of PerMaTa, on 17 March 2022.
25. Confirmed by the author in discussions with the Ministry of Health and PerMaTa members on 10 September 2018.
26. For example, PerMaTa South Sulawesi is currently actively utilizing the radio as a tool to promote accurate knowledge and understanding in regard to leprosy.
27. Email interview with Mr. Al Kadri, vice chairman of PerMaTa, on 17 March 2022.
28. Email interview with Mr. Tesfaye Tadesse, managing director of ENAPAL, on 20 March 2022.
29. Email interview with Mr. Tesfaye Tadesse, managing director of ENAPAL, on 20 March 2022.
30. Email interview with Mr. Amar Timalsina on 18 March 2022.
31. Email interview with Mr. Kofi Nyarko on 17 March 2022.
32. The issues to be discussed at the Global Forum were determined based on the topics for consideration at the three regional conferences that had been held previously in Africa (February 2019), Asia (March 2019) and Central America (March 2019).
33. "Summary, Conclusions and Recommendations—Global Forum of People's Organizations on Hansen's Disease in Manila, 7–10 September, 2019", https://www.shf.or.jp/en/information/6813 (accessed 27 December 2021).
34. "2nd Global Forum of People's Organizations on Hansen's Disease November 6–8, 2022, Hyderabad, India—Conclusions and Recommendations", https://sasakawaleprosyinitiative.org/latest-updates/initiative-news/2971/ (accessed 12 March 2023).
35. Resolution adopted by Human Rights Council on 12 August 2010 (A/HRC/RES/15/30), p. 4.
36. World Health Organization, Regional Office for South-East Asia, *Global Leprosy Strategy 2016–2020: Accelerating towards a leprosy-free world* (New Delhi: World Health Organization, 2001).
37. World Health Organization, Regional Office for South-East Asia, *Towards Zero Leprosy: Global Leprosy (Hansen's disease) Strategy 2021–2030* (New Delhi: World Health Organization, 2021).
38. UN Social Development Network, "Empowerment: What does it mean to you?" https://www.un.org/esa/socdev/ngo/outreachmaterials/empowerment-booklet.pdf (accessed 17 March 2022).

6. WHY PUBLIC AWARENESS MUST BE PROMOTED: ROLE OF THE WHO GOODWILL AMBASSADOR FOR LEPROSY ELIMINATION

1. *WHO Special Ambassador's Newsletter*, no. 1, Sasakawa Memorial Health Foundation, April 2003. https://www.leprosy-information.org/resource/who-goodwill-ambassadors-newsletter-elimination-leprosy (accessed 3 July 2023).

2. *WHO Special Ambassador's Newsletter*, no. 2, Sasakawa Memorial Health Foundation, June 2003. https://www.leprosy-information.org/resource/who-goodwill-ambassadors-newsletter-elimination-leprosy.

3. Yohei Sasakawa, *Making the Impossible Possible: My Work for Leprosy Elimination and Human Rights* (Tokyo: Kousakusha, 2021; London: Hurst, 2023), pp. 55.

4. Forum 2000 website, https://www.forum2000.cz/en/homepage (accessed 3 July 2023).

5. Sasakawa, *Making the Impossible Possible*, pp. 59–63.

6. Forum 2000, Shared Concern Initiative, "Human Rights and Leprosy", February 2011, https://www.forum2000.cz/en/human-rights-and-leprosy (accessed 3 July 2023).

7. Original articles are included in Yohei Sasakawa, *My Struggle against Leprosy* (Tokyo: Festina Lente Japan, 2019), pp. 159–226.

8. "The Global Appeal", The Nippon Foundation website, https://www.nippon-foundation.or.jp/en/what/projects/leprosy/appeal (accessed 3 July 2023).

9. The Japanese version of the Global Appeal 2006 announcement.

10. "Global Appeal 2006", The Nippon Foundation website, https://www.nippon-foundation.or.jp/en/what/projects/leprosy/appeal/2006 (accessed 3 July 2023).

11. "International Gandhi Award for Yohei Sasakawa", The Nippon Foundation Press Release, 12 April 2007.

12. "Mahatma Gandhi", ILA History of Leprosy website. https://leprosyhistory.org/database/person7 (accessed 3 July 2023).

13. Tony Gould, *Don't Fence Me In: From Curse to Cure: Leprosy in Modern Times* (London: Bloomsbury Publishing, 2005), https://www.ncbi.nlm.nih.gov/pmc/articles/PMC558396/ (accessed 3 July 2023).

14. Alec Jordan, "The 'Mahatma Gandhi of Japan' continues his battle against leprosy", *Tokyo Weekender*, 11 April 2017, https://www.tokyoweekender.com/Japan-life/news-and-opinion/the-mahatma-gandhi-of-japan-continues-his-battle-against-leprosy/ (accessed 3 July 2023).

15. "Gandhi Peace Prize for the years 2015, 2016, 2017 and 2018 announced", DD News, 17 January 2019, https://www.ddnews.gov.in/people/gandhi-peace-prize-years-2015-2016-2017-and-2018-announced (accessed 3 July 2023).

16. "Global Appeal 2013 to End Stigma and Discrimination Against People Affected by Leprosy", The Nippon Foundation website, https://www.nippon-foundation.or.jp/en/what/projects/leprosy/appeal/2013 (accessed 3 July 2023).

17. WHO Goodwill Ambassador's Newsletter for the Elimination of Leprosy (February 2013, No. 60): https://www.leprosy-information.org/resource/who-goodwill-ambassadors-newsletter-elimination-leprosy.

18. "Sasakawa Wins IBA Rule of Law Award for Efforts to End Leprosy Discrimination", The Nippon Foundation Press Release, October 2014, https://kyodonewsprwire.jp/release/201410234864 (accessed 3 July 2023).

19. Geoff Warne, "Eliminating discriminatory laws", *WHO Goodwill Ambassador's Leprosy Bulletin*, no. 105, September 2021, p. 3.

20. Annual thematic reports: Special Rapporteur on discrimination against persons with leprosy (Report A/76/148), https://www.ohchr.org/EN/Issues/Leprosy/Pages/Reports.aspx (accessed 3 July 2023).

21. "'THINK LEPROSY NOW': Global Appeal 2015", The Nippon Foundation website, https://www.nippon-foundation.or.jp/en/what/projects/leprosy/ga2015 (accessed 3 July 2023).

22. "Health and Human Rights Award", https://www.icn.ch/what-we-do/awards/health-and-human-rights-award/ (accessed 3 July 2023).

23. International Council of Nurses Health and Human Rights Award Press Release, June 2016.

24. "IPU helps to combat discrimination against people affected by leprosy", 31 January 2017. https://www.ipu.org/news/news-in-brief/2017–01/ipu-helps-combat-discrimination-against-people-affected-leprosy (accessed 3 July 2023).

25. "A Handbook for Parliamentarians: Eliminating Discrimination Against Persons Affected By Leprosy and Their Families" (2017). https://sasakawaleprosyinitiative.org/wp/wp-content/uploads/2022/05/A-Handbook-for-Parliamentarians.pdf (accessed 3 July 2023).

26. Diversity & Equal Opportunity Centre for Disabled Peoples' International, "Inclusion of People Affected by Leprosy in Disabled People's [sic] International: Report of the Baseline Study" (May 2014).

27. "Honoured to Be Part of the Struggle", *WHO Goodwill Ambassador's Newsletter*, no. 36, February 2009, p. 3.

28. "A Date with the Dalai Lama", *WHO Goodwill Ambassador's Newsletter*, no. 58, October 2012, p. 3.

29. *Ibid.*

30. Letters from Yohei Sasakawa to Pope Francis of 13 June 2013; 10 October 2013; 15 July 2014.

31. Interfaith Appeal to Eliminate Discrimination, https://www.nippon-foundation.or.jp/en/news/articles/2016/20160627–21038.html.

32. International Symposium, Vatican City, 9–10 June 2016, Conclusions and Recommendations. https://www.nippon-foundation.or.jp/media/archives/2018/en/news/articles/2016/img/32/7.pdf (accessed 3 July 2023).

33. Pope Francis, Angelus; St. Peter's Square, Sunday, 29 January 2017. https://

www.vatican.va/content/francesco/en/angelus/2017/documents/papa-fran-
cesco_angelus_20170129.html (accessed 3 July 2023).

34. Message from the Prefect of the Dicastery for Promoting Integral Human Development for the 64th World Leprosy Day, 28 January 2017. https://press.vatican.va/content/salastampa/en/bollettino/pubblico/2017/01/28/170128a.html (accessed 3 July 2023).

35. Message from the Prefect of the Dicastery for Promoting Integral Human Development for the 65th World Leprosy Day, 28 January 2018. https://press.vatican.va/content/salastampa/en/bollettino/pubblico/2018/01/28/180128a.html (accessed 3 July 2023).

36. Pope calls for united effort in fight against leprosy. https://www.vaticannews.va/en/pope/news/2021–01/pope-calls-for-united-effort-in-fight-against-leprosy.html (accessed 3 July 2023).

37. Message of the Prefect of the Dicastery for Promoting Integral Human Development on the occasion of the 68th World Leprosy Day, 31 January 2021. https://press.vatican.va/content/salastampa/en/bollettino/pubblico/2021/01/31/210131a.html; https://www.catholicnewsagency.com/tags/3402/leprosy (accessed 3 July 2023).

7. LEPROSY CONTROL IN THE POST-ELIMINATION ERA

1. P. Heyman, C. Cochez and M. Hukić, *The English Sweating Sickness: Out of Sight, Out of Mind?*, Acta Med. Acad. 47(1) (May 2019), pp. 102–16, doi: 10.5644/ama2006–124.221.

2. W. R. Dowdle, "The principles of disease elimination and eradication", *Bulletin of the World Health Organization* 76 (Suppl. 2) (1998), pp. 22–5.

3. P. Klepac, C. J. E. Metcalf, A. R. McLean and K. Hampson, "Towards the end-game and beyond: complexities and challenges for the elimination of infectious diseases", *Phil. Trans. R. Soc. B*, 368 (2013), 20120137, http://dx.doi.org/10.1098/rstb.2012.0137 (accessed 3 July 2023).

4. World Health Organization, *Ending the neglect to attain the Sustainable Development Goals: a road map for neglected tropical diseases 2021–2030* (Geneva: World Health Organization, 2020). Licence: CC BY-NC-SA 3.0 IGO Cataloguing-in-Publication.

5. Yohei Sasakawa, *No Matter Where the Journey Takes Me: One Man's Quest for a Leprosy-Free World* (London: Hurst, 2019).

6. "Ambassador's Message: Nepal marks elimination", *WHO Goodwill Ambassador's Newsletter*, no. 42, February 2010.

7. "Ambassador's Message: No Shame in Increased Case Numbers", *WHO Goodwill Ambassador's Newsletter*, no. 74, June 2015.

8. C. R. Filha, J. S. Silva, M. Virmond and V. L. G. Andrade, "Capacity building of primary care professionals by in-service in a multidisciplinary approach involving clinical leprosy, disability prevention and social mobilization—Bangkok

Declaration Special Fund Project Brazil", in Abstracts of the 20th International Leprosy Congress, International Convention Center, Manila, 10–13 September 2019.

9. World Health Organization, Regional Office for South-East Asia, Comprehensive Evaluation of Special Projects Bangkok Declaration Special Fund (BDSF) and Special Fund for Extraordinary circumstances (SFEC), 2021, Draft Report.

10. I. Mathauer and I. Imhoff, "Health worker motivation in Africa: the role of non-financial incentives and human resource management tools", *Human Resources for Health* 4, article 24 (2006).

11. P. Zurn, L. Dolea and B. Stilwell, *Nurse retention and recruitment: developing a motivated workforce* (Geneva: ICN, 2005).

12. D. F. C. Cordioli *et al.*, "Occupational stress and engagement in primary health care workers", *Revista Brasileira de Enfermagem* [online] 72(6) (2019), pp. 1580–1587. https://doi.org/10.1590/0034–7167–2018–0681; epub 21 October 2019: ISSN 1984–0446; https://doi.org/10.1590/0034–7167–2018–0681 (accessed 3 July 2023).

13. World Health Organization, "Report of the Global Forum on Elimination of Leprosy as a Public Health Problem, Geneva, Switzerland, 26 May 2006". Available at: https://apps.who.int/iris/handle/10665/69485 (accessed 3 July 2023).

14. "Ambassador's Message: Back to Brazil", *WHO Goodwill Ambassador's Newsletter*, no. 96, August 2019.

15. See "The Wheels of a Motorcycle", *WHO Goodwill Ambassador's Newsletter*, no. 80, June 2016.

16. Yohei Sasakawa, *No Matter Where the Journey Takes Me: One Man's Quest for a Leprosy-Free World* (London: Hurst, 2019).

17. Quoted in "A Study in Contrasts", *WHO Goodwill Ambassador's Newsletter*, no. 10, October 2004.

18. World Health Organization, *Ending the neglect to attain the Sustainable Development Goals: a road map for neglected tropical diseases 2021–2030* (Geneva: World Health Organization, 2020).

19. "No Shame in Increased Case Numbers", *WHO Goodwill Ambassador's Newsletter*, no. 74, June 2015.